PETER TYRER
ROGER HIGGS
GERALDINE STRATHDEE

Mental Health and Primary Care

A Changing Agenda

GASKELL & The Mental Health Foundation

Published by Gaskell on behalf of the Mental Health Foundation.
Gaskell is an imprint of the Royal College of Psychiatrists,
17 Belgrave Square, London SW1X 8PG

British Library Cataloguing-in-Publication Data

Tyrer, Peter
     Mental Health and Primary Care: Changing
     Agenda
     I. Title
     362.2

ISBN 0902241-53-2

Distributed in North America
by American Psychiatric Press, Inc.
ISBN 088048 619 8

Cover photograph by T. Shia.

Printed in Great Britain by Henry Ling Ltd., at the Dorset Press, Dorchester, Dorset

The authors

Peter Tyrer is Professor of Community Psychiatry at St Mary's Hospital Medical School, London

Roger Higgs is Professor of General Practice and Primary Care at King's College School of Medicine and Dentistry, London

Geraldine Strathdee is Consultant Psychiatrist in Rehabilitation and Community Care at the Maudsley Hospital, London

The Royal College of General Practitioners welcomes the publication of this book. The College was involved in planning the Conference at Cumberland Lodge that provided the forum at which many of these ideas were discussed. The College applauds the Mental Health Foundation's initiative in bringing together colleagues with different viewpoints to look at mental health and primary care, and discuss which areas should be given greater attention in both practical and research terms. I hope the contents of this book will help to raise awareness of the many important issues involved in delivering mental health care in the community among a wider audience than those who were able to attend the conference. The Royal College of General Practitioners supports the call for closer cooperation in this field, to which we hope this book will make a contribution.

Dr Mollie McBride
Honorary Secretary
Council of the Royal College of General Practitioners

Contents

KENSINGTON PALACE

There has never been a more important moment to bring together the skills and perspective of primary care and specialist mental health workers. We have begun to understand the widespread challenges to mental health, and to see how commonly such issues as homelessness, suicide, schizophrenia and the aftermath of disasters occur in the population.

The last decade has seen great advances in our appreciation of the inter-disciplinary needs of these problems. In response, we have seen progress in several directions - for instance, in the attachment of mental health workers to general practices; in holistic approaches to health care; increased user participation; advances in psychological and psychiatric research and improved treatment for those with a serious threat to their mental health.

However, such progress brings with it a realisation that whatever the importance of specialist teams, the challenge to mental health can never be addressed without all involved in health care working together to empower every potential patient, as far as can be, to care for their own mental health. In this, close co-operation and dialogue between psychiatrists and general practices are vital. As Patron of the Royal College of Psychiatrists and Past President of the Royal College of General Practitioners, I am proud to have witnessed such encouraging developments.

I, therefore, wholeheartedly endorse the work undertaken by those who attended the conference of which this book is a record, and the crucial support and encouragement of the Mental Health Foundation. It is a beginning, but a very important one.

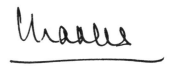

Introduction

The Mental Health Foundation has long been concerned about the importance of primary health care in the management of psychiatric illness. Ten years ago (Clare & Lader, 1981) it sponsored a seminal symposium on the subject and the subject has since achieved much greater prominence. Both psychiatrists and general practitioners have spread their wings to encompass much more than their original hospital and general practice territories, and as psychiatric teams have adopted multidisciplinary methods of working, the importance of liaison between psychiatry and primary care has assumed much greater importance. Approximately one in four of all psychiatrists now has regular clinical contacts with primary care services, and the importance of these services as the front line of psychiatric treatment has been emphasised by epidemiological studies, which demonstrate that ten times as many patients with psychiatric disorders of all kinds attend primary care services than those referred to psychiatrists (Goldberg & Huxley, 1992).

It may appear from published material that most of these initiatives have been developed by psychiatrists and that the general practitioner has been a passive partner. This would be a mistaken impression. Although the scene from general practice and psychiatry is not a panorama but a host of different perspectives, there has long been concern over the high prevalence of psychiatric problems in primary care and the most appropriate ways of treating them. These concerns have been highlighted in recent years following the closure of many mental hospitals and the general policy of moving towards community care for most people with mental illness.

Multidisciplinary working involves much more than medical input, and insufficient attention has sometimes been given to the contribution of the other members of both primary care and psychiatric teams. These include community psychiatric nurses, social workers – both generic and specialised – health visitors, district and practice nurses, occupational therapists, psychologists and counsellors. There is also a great amount of mental health care provided by voluntary organisations, notably MIND and the National Schizophrenia Fellowship, but many others provide care, and help to focus on deficiencies in policies and resources, both national and local.

This book stems from a conference on primary health care and psychiatric disorder held in Windsor, 19–21 July 1991, where around 50 delegates from general practice, psychiatry, and the voluntary sector met to discuss these issues. The format of the meeting was unusual. Instead of individual speakers presenting data or opinions from positions of authority, the main part of the conference consisted of small groups discussing the issues that confront all practitioners who treat mental health problems in primary care – people in acute crises, those abusing drugs, others with long-term and apparently intractable mental illness, those who attend the surgery frequently irrespective of any benefit, the special problems of black and ethnic minorities, and patients who are categorised as 'difficult to place'. Subsequently, similar small groups examined the possible solutions to each of these issues, including the possibilities for improved training in the special problems of mental illness in general practice, the best ways of collaboration between primary care and psychiatric teams, the role of users in mental health care, and the types of support needed for carers. This structure allowed a large number of questions and opinions to be expressed, which themselves generated others before the end of the meeting.

This book was stimulated by the conference, but is not a report of it. The Mental Health Foundation felt it was important to give a wider circulation to these questions and views, and also to suggest some answers, even if many of them could be regarded as speculative because there is so little information available to answer them. In any case, many of the questions raised can be answered only if the resources are available to investigate them, and the Mental Health Foundation has acknowledged the importance of this subject by setting up a new Projects Committee for Primary Care.

When information is limited, opinions are rife, and during the meeting in Windsor many were expressed. Although these could be discussed individually, there was a tendency for them to group into three, one each from primary care, psychiatry, and the voluntary sector. This is perhaps not surprising, as each area has a different input into mental health problems in primary care, concentrating its help on part of the population only. Sometimes the views of the three coincided, but more often they diverged. Rather than hide these divisions, we thought it better to expose them fully, because consensus solutions can be reached only if the divisions are fully acknowledged. So in this book we have recorded these differences frankly, and, indeed, have highlighted them by presenting the unabridged and unadulterated views of all. By bringing these into the open, the dangers are avoided of policy being decided by the most vocal or influential group at the expense of minorities.

In presenting these views, we are throwing down the gauntlet to clinicians, research workers, and managers in the health services. We ask a lot of questions and provide suggestions sometimes amounting to guidelines, but no definitive answers, apart from the need for resources to tackle these problems. At regular intervals in the text, we summarise some of the questions that need answering, once the financial resources are available to fund appropriate investigations. We believe we have set forth an agenda that needs to be addressed if community care for mental illness is to become a reality.

Fortunately, we are blessed in the UK in having a comprehensive system of primary care that, despite some fraying at the edges, is still the envy of the world. General practitioners and their colleagues in the primary care services are the gatekeepers to all of the services, including the mental health ones, even if there is some argument over what exactly constitutes a mental health problem. Critics of both the psychiatric and primary care services complain frequently of the ease with which psychiatric patients can slip through the net of follow-up and translate community care to community neglect. This need not be the case, because if psychiatric care services are appropriate the metaphor of slipping through the net is an inappropriate one. Such patients merely transfer from one type of care to another at a time when they no longer need the support of the institution and can continue with the resources available in primary care. The popular word to describe this transition is 'seamless', and although it is becoming hackneyed, this effortless transition from one type of care to another is the ideal that should be aimed for wherever possible.

We hope that the issues raised in this book will provoke and stimulate each of us, whatever our professional backgrounds, into considering these issues and at least looking at solutions. The outcome is literally an agenda: a set of points for discussion and possible courses of action, but few prescriptions or instructions.

The Mental Health Foundation is pleased to have facilitated this exchange of views and would like to thank all the delegates who took part, as well as Cynthia Fletcher, Senior Projects Officer of the Foundation, and her staff for organising the conference so efficiently. We should also like to thank Brice Pitt, Clive Evers, Paul Freeling, Linda Gask, Elena Garralda, David Goldberg, Helen Hally, John Horder, Anthony Kendrick, Michael King, Mollie McBride, Alistair Macdonald, Parimala Moodley, John Reed, Meredith Robson and André Tylee for reviewing sections of this book and for their constructive comments, and to Ann Tyrer and Marie Jayakody for their secretarial help. We look forward to another meeting in ten years' time in which we hope to report that many of the challenges set forth in this book have been taken up, investigated, and solved. This will be made much more likely if we are able to obtain the resources necessary to fund these projects. The Mental Health Foundation promises to play its part in securing these; we hope others will follow.

Peter Tyrer, Roger Higgs and Geraldine Strathdee
and Robert Loder on behalf of the Primary Care Working Party,
Mental Health Foundation

1 What are we trying to achieve?

Nearly one in four patients seen in general practice suffer from some form of psychiatric illness (Ormel & Giel, 1990) and almost all patients discharged from psychiatric hospitals receive at least some part of their treatment from the general practitioner (GP) or primary care team. As the Mental Health Foundation has noted, 5.9 million people living in the community in the UK have a mental illness, yet only 60 000 are hospital in-patients (Mental Health Foundation, 1990). As primary care services in the UK are universal (although not everyone is registered with a GP) it illustrates that most patients with mental illness (and their relatives) are likely to be in contact with their GP or another member of the primary care team. So however one looks at primary care psychiatry, it is impossible to avoid the conclusion that if there are problems in the care of this population they are likely to be important in national terms because they are so widespread.

It is possible to be overwhelmed by the size of this problem and retreat into discussion of epidemiological terms such as prevalence, incidence and case identification without considering how much individual suffering is caused by mental illness and how each 'episode' of mental illness, however categorised by those who need to collect statistics, has its own unique qualities that make it specific to that person and to his or her carers.

We also need to remind ourselves that all of us are liable to suffer mental illness and, despite the uniqueness of each experience, similar distress can be suffered by almost anybody. If we refer to psychiatric patients, in whatever setting, as 'cases', we are in danger of stigmatising mental illness by setting boundaries between it and allegedly normal mental health. Nevertheless, we have to demarcate those suffering an episode of mental illness at any one time from those who are not, and the word 'case' has the merit of easy understanding. Where we use it in this text we are doing so as a convenient shorthand, as each is an exemplar of a much larger group of patients in distress who are seeking help or for whom help is being sought on their behalf.

We also need to be aware that the suffering of patients with mental illness cannot be discussed in isolation from its setting. One of the reasons why the Mental Health Foundation is concentrating its attention on psychiatry in primary care is that primary care is generally more sensitive to setting and cannot externalise mental illness in the way that hospitals sometimes can. It is quite possible for psychiatric hospitals to operate as though they were large casualty departments, with emergencies being brought in at unpredictable intervals (most psychiatric admissions are emergencies), treated for their immediate symptoms and problems (mainly abnormal behaviour), and then launched into the world again. This may seem like a caricature, but when staff work entirely in hospital it is easy to fall into this way of thinking. Many staff based in institutions honestly deny such attitudes when directly alleged because much of these attitudes are so entrenched in the structures of their daily professional life that they are seldom acknowledged, never mind questioned.

While it could be argued that this limited horizon is appropriate for a hospital-based service, it is not appropriate for a comprehensive service. When the hospital system of care attempts to decide on the after-care of its patients in what is often a vacuum of knowledge about community and primary care services, it is to be expected that their plans will be unrealistic and uninformed, and will quickly go awry.

General practitioners are in a different position from hospital psychiatrists. They deal with all forms of illness, in most of which there will be a mixture of mental and physical components. Deciding which deserves more emphasis in the time constraints of general practice requires almost superhuman skill, and success may not always be achieved first time. The relationship between the GP and the patient is critical, and as it lasts, in most cases, much longer than the relationship between hospital doctor and patient, it is important for it to be based on trust and mutual respect. This can often can be difficult to maintain, particularly with patients who become too dominant or demanding, and as GPs have no institutional options to fall back on, they often have to struggle with these difficulties alone or share them with other members of the primary care team. When referring patients to psychiatrists it is difficult for the GP to put these problems over in a way that is understandable and immediately appreciated, because in general the hospital psychiatrist looks at the issues from a different perspective. However, both are trying to achieve a combination of understanding, comfort, clinical improvement and coping ability, and improving the links between psychiatry and primary care should help to construct a common language.

To illustrate some of these more complex and personal issues, in this chapter we describe two cases that illustrate the extremes (hence the alpha and omega) of good and bad practice in the community care of mental illness, and discuss their implications. These raise many issues concerning quality of care, communication, coordination between professionals, and concern. There are dangers in generalising from single cases, but few would disagree that we need to aim for targets that allow alpha care to become routine rather than exceptional. The following accounts are of real patients, but small changes have been made to conceal their identities.

Case 1

Mrs Alpha was a 49-year-old divorcee who had been seeing her GP for four years with problems over close personal relationships. She came from a strict family; after rebelling against this degree of control in adolescence, she had embarked on a passionate affair, leading to a marriage which had failed. Among the reasons for the marital break-down was Mrs Alpha's volatile temperament. At times she was optimistic and felt she could achieve almost anything, whereas at others she became doubting, suspicious of others and gloomy about the future.

She consulted a GP originally over symptoms of anxiety and depression. He considered that these were likely to be related to a relationship which she had started four years earlier which was getting into difficulties in exactly the same way as her first marriage. He felt that tranquilliser and antidepressant medication was inappropriate in this context and arranged to see her at short intervals over six months. After this time he felt it appropriate to refer her to his practice nurse who had undertaken courses in counselling and was experienced in dealing with problems of relationships, particularly those of a sexual nature. She was seen over the next three years by the practice nurse, who regularly reported her progress to the GP. Considerable progress was achieved. In particular, it appeared that Mrs Alpha had never been able to shake off entirely the expectation of extremely high standards instilled by her upbringing. She came to appreciate gradually that if these standards were excessive she was bound to fail when trying to achieve them. She had also continued to feel that she was basically a failure in her parents' eyes because she had gone against their wishes in pursuing the relationship that led to her marriage. When the marriage subsequently failed this not only vindicated her parents' philosophy but made the fault irredeemable.

As a consequence of developing these insights Mrs Alpha's current relationship with a divorced man of the same age improved. The couple decided on a more permanent relationship and decided to live together before considering marriage. Cohabitation had previously been considered out of the question by Mrs Alpha; her parents had instilled in her the view that it was a sin.

However, despite these many improvements Mrs Alpha continued to have swings of mood. She sometimes considered herself to be unworthy of her new lover and was convinced that he would abandon her in favour of a younger, more attractive woman. At these times she could not be reassured by him or her practice nurse and was close to despair. At other times she became expansive, more sexually active, and sometimes embarrassed her lover with her extravagant displays of affection in public places. Matters reached a crisis when she was unfaithful to her lover and compared his sexual prowess unfavourably with that of her new paramour. She was irritable and hypercritical of his small foibles, such as his attachment to his pet cat, and some of her remarks were deeply wounding.

The practice nurse and the GP discussed these problems at some length and the possibility that Mrs Alpha had a form of more serious mental disturbance was discussed. It was decided that Mrs Alpha should be asked whether she would consider seeing a psychiatrist (she had never done so before) and the subject was gently introduced at her next counselling session. At first she was extremely angry that for the first time in her life mental illness of a more formal nature was being implied (her problems had never been described as mental illness before) and was understandably ambivalent about psychiatric referral. Her GP contacted the psychiatrist and explained these difficulties by telephoning immediately after sending the referral and the psychiatrist offered to see the patient at the GP's surgery if this was likely to be more acceptable. Mrs Alpha she was quite happy with this arrangement, but asked for the counsellor to be present at the interview.

After assessment the psychiatrist felt that there was sufficient information to consider a diagnosis of (bipolar) manic–depressive psychosis, even though the episodes of affective disturbance were not severe. He felt it was appropriate to consult other informants, and Mrs Alpha agreed to the psychiatrist seeing her brother to discuss whether her mood swings had been present over a long period. A subsequent interview with Mrs Alpha's brother established that she had had her mood swings since late adolescence and, more significantly, that one of her uncles suffered from what appeared to be a classic form of manic–depressive illness and subsequently died in a psychiatric hospital. This information had been kept from the family because Mrs Alpha's parents felt so ashamed about it; her brother had found out about it independently.

The combination of persistent mood disturbance with both manic and depressive phases, together with evidence of a family history of a similar disorder, led the psychiatrist to make a formal diagnosis of bipolar affective psychosis. After discussion with Mrs Alpha, later reinforced with the GP and counsellor in a joint meeting, Mrs Alpha agreed to take lithium in the form of its carbonate salt for at least two years in the first instance, to see whether the mood swings would be attenuated.

The GP agreed to monitor the lithium dosage and the practice nurse (in one of her other roles) was involved in regular venepunctures and monitoring of the serum lithium levels. After a year on treatment with no further episodes of depressive or manic disturbance it was clear that the therapy was beneficial. Apart from some increase in the frequency of micturition, lithium produced no abnormal effects and annual checks of thyroid function were normal. Mrs Alpha then agreed to continue treatment for a further five years and is currently taking this. One of the main consequences of the improvement in her mood was that her relationship with her cohabitee became much closer and the couple are now married.

The case of Mrs Alpha demonstrates several cardinal features of good primary care and liaison with psychiatrists. Firstly, the primary care team, in the form of the GP and his practice nurse/counsellor, are clearly in the driving seat throughout the period of care described. They understand Mrs Alpha's problem and deal with it appropriately until a crisis brings to the fore an issue which, after proper discussion, leads to a request for further help. It is only at this point that the psychiatrist is contacted and, as soon as advice has been recommended from this source, the primary care team is able to take on most of the clinical responsibility again.

Secondly, the wishes and needs of Mrs Alpha have been sensitively considered throughout. It might be more accurate to say that she is in the driving seat, as it is only by improving her self-confidence and trust that so much progress was made in understanding the key problems of the initial presentation. Her reluctance about seeing a psychiatrist was overcome by assessment at the GP's surgery together with her counsellor.

Thirdly, the psychiatrist was consulted at an appropriate time, when there were many forms of management available apart from admission to hospital (all too often the only option when a patient is referred in a severe crisis). He was able, because of all the information obtained and the work carried out by the GP and practice nurse, to come to an adequate assessment of the diagnostic options, which were finalised after seeing Mrs Alpha's brother. He was being used for his specific skills, and not asked, in the unspoken message of many referrals from primary care, "Please take this impossible patient off my hands for a bit; I can't cope with her any longer". The referral was coordinated and clear, and the joint consultation in general practice ensured that this clarity and precision was maintained. The benefit to Mrs Alpha needs no further emphasis.

Before we become complacent it is necessary to move on quickly to the opposite end of the spectrum, where the failures of good liaison, like many failures in medicine, tend to attract more attention than the successes.

Case 2

Mr Omega was a man of 22. He was born in London but both his parents came from Barbados, in the West Indies. Although his early life was reasonably happy his parents were increasingly in conflict by the time he became an adolescent and separated three years ago. Mr Omega was closer to his mother and lived with her after the separation. He did reasonably well at school and worked as a car mechanic after leaving full-time education. He first became unwell at the age of 19. His parents noticed that he had become more withdrawn and often seemed to be in a world of his own. Later he became convinced that he had been selected by God to save the world from corruption and that his body was merely an agent of God's will. He became aggressive when these beliefs were challenged and after he assaulted his father the police were called. He was subsequently admitted to hospital compulsorily, at first under Section 136, and subsequently Section 2, of the Mental Health Act 1983.

He improved quickly in hospital and was discharged on oral antipsychotic drugs as he preferred these to depot injections. While in hospital he had been dispossessed of his flat, and so he stayed with his mother for a short time after leaving hospital, before getting another flat close by. He failed to keep out-patient appointments after two months, but his GP, who had received only a discharge letter after he had first left hospital (giving details of his out-of-date address), was not informed. A community nurse had been asked by the consultant to see Mr Omega and, after some difficulty, she eventually was able to contact him. At this stage he was beginning to get unwell again and refused to take medication. The community nurse decided she could do nothing further, reported this to the consultant, and contact ceased. The GP was not informed about this decision.

Over the next four months Mr Omega continued to deteriorate. As by now he was living in his own flat he had less contact with his parents and became even more withdrawn. He again developed grandiose ideas about changing the world and having supernatural powers. When he attempted to stop a police car to take him on one of his 'missions' he was at first arrested and, when his mental state was seen to be abnormal, was taken to the casualty department and subsequently admitted to a psychiatric hospital, again on a compulsory order.

He was discharged after two months, but a *laissez-faire* attitude was taken about the previous relapse and it was assumed that nothing further could be done to change matters apart from strongly encouraging him to maintain contact after being discharged. He agreed to do this and was seen by a community nurse before he left hospital. After discharge the community nurse continued to see him and provided medication but he would not attend clinics and sometimes it was difficult to see him regularly. After six months the community nurse left, and the case load was passed to another nurse. The previous problems encountered with Mr Omega were not made clear and he was sent an appointment to be seen at a follow-up clinic run by the community nurse. Again no communication was made to the GP. Not surprisingly, Mr Omega failed to attend this clinic and was crossed off the list of the new community nurse after he had failed two other appointments.

Three months later Mr Omega again relapsed, which was entirely predictable on the basis of his history. On this occasion he remained in the community for eight months before being admitted to hospital compulsorily under similar circumstances to his other admissions. On this occasion, however, his flat was repossessed after admission because he had not paid rent for the previous six months. By the time of discharge he was homeless and was accommodated in bed-and-breakfast accommodation outside the catchment area of the psychiatric hospital.

This case history is not exceptional – would that it was – and illustrates several of the failures in care that can result from poor GP–psychiatric liaison that are worth examining in turn. The initial failure of the family to contact the GP at an early stage of Mr Omega's illness (not in itself an indication of poor liaison) meant that he presented as an emergency to the psychiatric services. The cycle was then established of periods of mental health and active care alternating with steady deterioration in symptoms and functioning associated with no care, leading inevitably to a compulsory emergency admission. However, once in hospital the primary care services could have been more closely involved in the after-care plans. As it happened, the GP received only a standard discharge letter and apparently had no role in after-care.

The after-care provided was limited and almost entirely hospital based; once Mr Omega defaulted on his out-patient appointments everything depended on the community psychiatric nurse. No one appeared to take responsibility for this after-care (i.e. there was no care manager) and there were no regular reviews of his progress by the professionals involved. This is an unsatisfactory state of affairs, as a community nurse cannot expect to be monitoring patients in isolation. At least in a case such as this, in which integration of care had already been shown to be difficult, there should be additional support from other professionals, with a clear plan of action ready to be implemented when contact with the patient is lost. In addition, long-term medication for every patient should be monitored by either the psychiatrist or the GP, as dosage requirements may change. With only one weak link binding Mr Omega to the psychiatric team it was not surprising that when this link temporarily broke (by the departure of the community nurse) it was not possible to re-establish it with the new community nurse. Mr Omega therefore dropped out of care and deterioration was more marked subsequently because his parents no longer monitored him so closely.

During his slow deterioration after stopping medication Mr Omega received no after-care whatsoever and had no contact with any part of the voluntary or statutory services. Although this can often not be prevented in the first episode of a schizophrenic illness, there is no justification for it being repeated. The failure to maintain contact with Mr Omega after he defaulted from treatment on the second occasion should have set the alarm bells ringing in the psychiatric team, so that further efforts would be made to establish contact again and engage him in some sort of therapy, not necessarily pharmacological. Even if this were refused, it is appropriate for the services to maintain a monitoring role so that admission is not left to the last possible moment, when patients are often dangerous to others as well as a serious risk to themselves. Because of the delay in establishing care again there was a real danger that Mr Omega would lose his flat and become homeless after discharge from hospital on the final occasion.

Research questions
- What are the most effective ways of distinguishing between good and poor psychiatry in general practice?
- Would the allocation of a care manager to all psychiatric patients before discharge improve after-care?

- For which groups, if any, should the psychiatric services retain long-term primary responsibility?
- When is it appropriate for a primary care professional to be involved in the discharge of patients from psychiatric hospitals?

Conclusions

In situations like this there is a tendency for territorial arguments to take over from concern for patient care. The psychiatric services often argue that local authority social services are deficient in monitoring patients who are discharged without supervision from in-patient care, but equally, the local authority services can complain that the mental health after-care services are deficient when patients who are in active care fail to be followed up because they default from their appointments. This type of argument is fruitless and hinders good liaison, and while ostensibly being carried out in the interests of patient care is far more often used to justify inactivity or as an attempt to obtain extra resources. If services are sensitive to the needs and wishes of their users the problems of territory do not arise.

Mental health services differ from other medical ones in that they also have a function in protecting society from the effects of mental illness, and so sometimes the users' wishes have to be over-ruled, but this does not mean they should be ignored. With Mrs Alpha the wishes and aims of patient, primary care team and psychiatrist were all in harmony; with Mr Omega they were not so much discordant as disconnected. 'Out of sight, out of mind' is so often true with mental illness. We do not search for many lost patients whom we know to be unwell; we do not care for those who seem not to appreciate what we have to offer; and we do not anticipate danger even when the signs are there for all to see. Until we do, Mr Omega will have many fellow sufferers at the bottom of the alphabet.

It could be argued that Mrs Alpha and Mr Omega are not fair examples as they are not equivalent, with one presenting through the emergency services and the other through the GP, one with good networks and the other with poor ones, and so on. These differences are acknowledged but they are not fundamental ones. As a postscript it is worth adding that Mr Omega, who was registered with a single-handed GP, is now with a group practice with a practitioner who has a special interest in mental health problems. He attends the clinic regularly for his antipsychotic drug prescriptions and, on the occasions he forgets and does not respond to reminders, a community mental health service is contacted and he is visited at home. He is much more settled and on a substantially lower dose than formally. He is moving up the alphabet!

2 How big is the problem?

As indicated in Chapter 1, most psychiatric disorder, both major and minor, is seen by professionals outside psychiatric hospitals. By far the largest proportion of these professionals are GPs and so what happens to psychiatric disorder in general practice is of fundamental importance. Fortunately we now know much more about this subject since psychiatric epidemiology in general practice has become an established discipline, stimulated by the pioneering work of Michael Shepherd and his colleagues begun in 1959 (Shepherd *et al*, 1959) and expanded dramatically since (Shepherd *et al*, 1966, 1986). The sheer volume of psychiatric disorder seen in general practice is shown by the figures of Goldberg & Huxley (1980, 1992) which show the prevalence of psychiatric disorder in each of five different population levels, ranging from the community at one extreme to psychiatric in-patients at the other (Table 1). The ratio between those attending primary care facilities and those being seen as psychiatric in-patients has increased from 38.3 in 1980 to 40.3 in 1992, but over the same time the numbers seen by the mental health services as a whole have increased by 28%, so illustrating the move away from hospital towards community care.

It is clear from the figures that the large number of people who attend primary care with mental disorder is of key importance in the psychiatric services. Even so, it would be wrong to infer from these that patients in primary care have the same level of illness (equivalent morbidity) as those in hospital care, and the figures do not explain how patients pass through the filters to the different parts of the psychiatric services.

In Fig. 1 the proportions of patients coming to psychiatric care from five countries which are relatively well resourced in mental health services (England, Portugal, Spain, Czechoslovakia, and Cuba) are summarised. The study, carried out with the support of the World Health Organization, recorded the details of all patients receiving a new episode of psychiatric care in a calendar month (Gater *et al*, 1991). The importance

TABLE 1

The five levels and four filters of psychiatric care

		Annual period prevalence rates: 1000/year
Level 1	Community	260–315
	First filter (illness behaviour)	
Level 2	Total mental morbidity (attenders in primary care)	230
	Second filter (ability to detect disorder)	
Level 3	Conspicuous psychiatric morbidity (detected by doctors)	101.5
	Third filter (referral to mental illness services)	
Level 4	Total morbidity (mental illness services)	23.5
	Fourth filter (admission to psychiatric beds)	
Level 5	Psychiatric in-patients	5.71

Reproduced with permission of Goldberg & Huxley (1992).

of the GP in the referral process is clear: by far the largest proportion of patients referred to psychiatrists come from this source. In the English component of the study, carried out in Manchester, Gater & Goldberg (1991) found that 63% of patients came directly from the GP but, interestingly, that hospital doctors referred 28% of the patients, a larger proportion than in the other centres. Examination of the intervals between referral and assessment indicated that the filter process was a relatively fast one. On average, the GP managed their patients for three weeks before referring to the psychiatrist and there was a two-week interval before the patient was seen (Gater & Goldberg, 1991).

The international study, which was carried out in a total of 11 countries, also showed that in the countries poorly provided with mental health services, such as Pakistan, India and Indonesia, pathways were dominated by direct referrals from the community to the psychiatric services. A similar referral process is found in the US, termed 'the American by-pass' by Goldberg & Huxley (1980), indicating that national affluence is not the only factor in operation here. However one interprets these data, and they cannot be used to compare the quality of the services in the different countries, they show that in those countries where there are many physicians in primary care the referral process of patients with mental illness is dominated by the GP.

Of course, these data refer only to the relatively small number of individuals who pass from primary care to secondary care. The study did not examine the large numbers of patients who are managed in primary

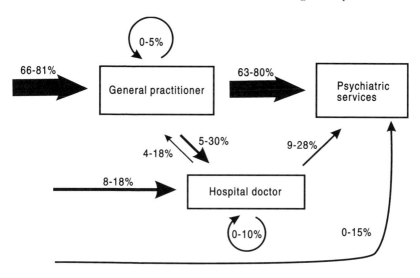

Fig. 1. Pathways to psychiatric care in five countries (from Gater et al, 1991). The community is shown on the left, and the size of each arrow indicates the relative importance of each pathway. Numbers shown are percentages of those receiving care from the psychiatric services over a calendar month. (Reproduced by permission of Gater et al and Psychological Medicine)

care, who cover the whole range of mental illness, and who are not referred because the GP has both recognised the nature of the illness and feels competent to deal with it successfully.

Nevertheless, it is again important to stress that although 230 per 1000 attenders in primary care per year have some mental disorder, this group of disorders should not be regarded as equivalent to those seen at other levels. Not surprisingly, most sufferers from mental illness in primary care have less handicap and less severe symptoms than psychiatric in-patients. In general, what are commonly described as the major psychoses (mainly affective psychoses and schizophrenia) constitute by far the largest proportion of those in psychiatric in-patient beds, whereas those in primary care are predominantly suffering from depressive and anxiety disorders, together with patients suffering what are now described under the cumbersome heading of 'somatoform disorders'. In these conditions patients present with somatic symptoms and attribute these to physical disorder. On examination, often reinforced by investigations because of the doctor's uncertainty or the patient's insistence, no physical disorder is found, but the symptoms do show a characteristic pattern that justifies the description of a psychiatric disorder using current classifications (Bridges & Goldberg, 1985).

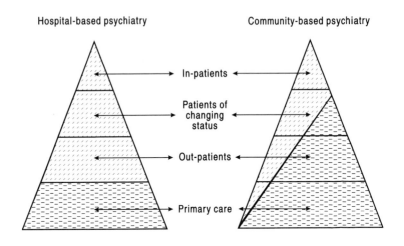

Fig. 2. The interface between general practice and psychiatry in hospital and community psychiatry (▨ psychiatric service; ▤ general practice service) (from Tyrer, 1986, and reproduced by permission of the Journal of the Royal College of General Practitioners)

However, the view commonly held in psychiatric practice for some years, that most of the mental disorders in primary care are too minor for psychiatrists to be concerned about and can be dealt with quite simply by the GP, has never been apposite and is even less so now. Although such disorders in primary care are described as 'minor' or 'mild', they create considerable suffering and handicap and, because of their numbers, cost in the UK twice as much to treat as psychiatric in-patients (Croft-Jeffreys & Wilkinson, 1989).

In recent years the transfer of psychiatric patients, formerly in psychiatric hospitals for long periods, to various forms of community care has accelerated. Formerly, such patients were often permanent residents in mental hospitals and received all their care from the staff there. Now they are being discharged and placed in supervised hostels, independent accommodation or other institutions in which the primary care services are heavily involved. This does not mean that the filters between the different levels of care are breaking down, but there is a much wider interface between the primary care and psychiatric services now than there was a few years ago (Fig. 2).

Despite the size of the problem there are still surprisingly few resources devoted to the study of psychiatry in primary care. Over the last 20 years there has been a steady growth in the number of psychiatrists who have regular contacts with GPs in the form of clinics, regular liaison meetings or joint working arrangements (Strathdee & Williams, 1983; Pullen & Yellowlees, 1988; Kendrick *et al*, 1991). These figures suggest that currently approximately one in four of all psychiatrists have such contacts. What is most interesting about these figures is that they do not follow any directive from central government or health authorities but have come about from both the need to devolve and extend many of the psychiatric services that used to be confined to psychiatric hospitals, as well as a genuine wish to improve liaison. It also seems to have had benefits in reducing demands for in-patient care (Tyrer *et al*, 1984; Williams & Balestrieri, 1989). However, despite the merits of promoting local flexibility in working arrangements, the general impression of these services is that they are ad hoc developments that do not follow any defined plan or policy. There is a need for research to coordinate and evaluate the knowledge and experience obtained from these enterprises so that good models of collaboration can be recommended to others. However, because the disciplines concerned have differing visions of their priorities it is not always easy to unify them, and this reinforces the open format of this book. We need to make full allowance for these differences in planning services and undertaking research.

Much of the difference of opinion comes from the variation in training given to the professionals involved in the psychiatric services, training that shows little evidence of integration. There is also too much territoriality, a cumbersome but necessary word to describe the tendency of each discipline to mark out boundaries on the map of mental illness and make an independent province separated from the others. Far too much unnecessary time is spent in bureaucratic confrontation across these boundaries, instead of in helping our customers. Much of this conflict has a historical basis. For much of the last 200 years doctors have dominated the mental health professions, administratively, politically and clinically. It is hardly surprising that when each separate discipline has been allowed to break free from the influence of the medical profession it has preferred to carve out its own destiny instead of seeking active collaboration with its former masters. There is also a perfectly good reason why these disciplines should be separate from the medical profession. Each has a different knowledge base and pattern of training and, in several instances, a major difference in philosophy as well. All these handicap multidisciplinary working. Goldberg & Huxley (1992) offer some tart comments about the current state of mental health disciplines:

"The lack of unity of service has been accompanied by a rather narrow view of training by each profession. In England, clinical psychologists know very little about social psychiatry and epidemiology; social workers know very little about either psychology or the biological basis of mental disorders; and our psychiatrists all too often adopt either a narrowly biological approach to their subject, or an approach heavily emphasising dynamic psychiatry which is relatively uninfluenced by recent advances in either biological, or social psychiatry." (pp. 162–163)

If one is open to these difficulties they are more likely to be overcome than if they are forgotten or ignored.

Research questions
- Does greater understanding of psychological issues in primary care reduce the incidence of somatically orientated psychiatric (somatoform) disorder?
- What is preventing the majority of psychiatrists and GPs from active collaboration?
- Is there a place for common funding of mental health problems in primary care from which both GPs and psychiatric services can be supported?

The psychiatric viewpoint

The typical psychiatrist looks on general practice as an excellent system for separating the 'real' mentally ill patients from the remainder, who are often described by the offensive term the 'worried well'. (It is never made clear whether these people are worried because they are well or well because they only worry.) He (more frequently than she) is very satisfied with the GP acting as a filter between the many patients in the community who have mental symptoms and their own specialist services which deal with genuine mental illness. These disorders seen by GPs are recognised to be important but the apparent success of primary care teams in treating them without recourse to psychiatric referral suggests that the GPs are competent and require no further skills (apart from training to help them to recognise psychiatric illness more frequently) (Table 1). There are still many psychiatrists who believe strongly that most mental health problems seen by GPs are self-limiting and need no special expertise.

The psychiatrist often has a rough and ready definition of serious mental illnesses: they are conditions that need to be treated at some time by psychiatrists and in many instances require admission to hospital. These, in terms of the mental health services, can be represented as a boat (Fig. 3). A significant proportion, but always well under 50%, of the patients with major psychiatric morbidity have at least some regular contact with the psychiatric services, and only a minority are beneath the water and below the threshold of contact. Because of the move away from hospital care, an increasing proportion of psychiatric patients are

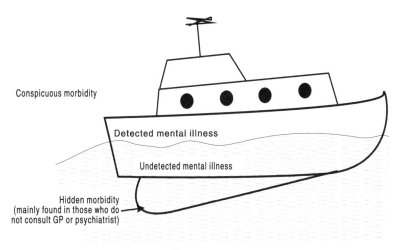

Conspicuous morbidity

Detected mental illness

Undetected mental illness

Hidden morbidity
(mainly found in those who do
not consult GP or psychiatrist)

Fig. 3. The recognition of major mental illness by psychiatrists

now treated at home or in other forms of community provision, and shared care between psychiatric and general practice teams is commonplace. There was a tendency in the past for patients with severe mental disorder, who commonly spent a large part of their lives in hospital, to have separate medical services and, when they turned up at the GP's surgery they were regarded as interlopers who really belonged to the psychiatric services. This view is of historical interest only but is still handicapping progress in some settings. Some GPs make it clear that they prefer patients with no psychiatric disorder because mental health problems are perceived as time consuming, difficult if not impossible to solve, and often show a predilection for difficult and odd personalities.

To enable attitudes to change, the psychiatrist realises that the GP needs more skills in dealing with major mental illness. To some extent this has already been anticipated in training programmes for general practice. All GPs go through a formal training scheme in different specialties, and 50% include hospital psychiatry in that scheme for at least six months. This attachment allows the developing GP both to see the types of illness that are seen by psychiatrists, as well the options for care available, and to discover which resources are available in psychiatric care and denied to the GP. This enables a much more informed view to be developed about the indications for referral.

Psychiatrists also need training in general practice. This has been formalised in some training programmes, particularly at St George's Hospital in London, and informal attachments take place in some other areas. However, we are not yet sure of the best form of such training, how it could be incorporated generally into the professional requirements of bodies such as the Royal College of Psychiatrists, at what point in the rotation should the attachment take place, and whether it should be a continuous attachment for, say, three to six months, or offered on a day-release basis.

Psychiatrists feel that they already provide quite a good service to GPs both on the ground, through expansion of primary care clinics, other forms of liaison (Creed & Marks, 1989), and in training, through their rotational schemes for trainees in general practice. Whether or not this is unduly complacent is difficult to tell; there is no doubt that general practice trainees now know more about major mental illness and its treatment in psychiatric units than they did in the past. The psychiatrist thinks this is important because it is only right for the GP when he/she makes a referral to the psychiatrist to know the kind of management that is likely to be given.

The general practice viewpoint

In recent years the GPs have increased in confidence in their ability to cope with psychiatric problems in primary care. This has come about partly because of better training but also from greater awareness of the advantages of continuity of care. A good GP realises that if he/she is able to cope with the psychiatric problems within primary care there will be advantages for all. Increasingly, too, GPs realise that psychiatrists have little to offer them in the care of the most common problems in general practice. Although some of the more severe forms of depression and anxiety are referred to psychiatrists, these account only for about one-sixth of the total (Fahy, 1974) and most of these disorders are treated by and large successfully by primary care throughout the UK.

What the GP wants is access to additional psychiatric resources that would help to keep the patient within primary care and allow the GP to take medical responsibility, or that gives some additional expertise and time which is not available from within the primary care team. The notion of psychiatrists visiting the general practice to give advice on how to treat patients in primary care has some merits but has a patronising quality to it. GPs are best at treating their own patients and when these are seen entirely in primary care it is hardly appropriate for the psychiatrist to speak with authority on the ideal management for such patients. Of course it may be necessary for the GP to call in a psychiatrist from time to time, but this is necessary only when patients need more intensive treatment or when there is a specific reason for the consultation rather than a wish to transfer care. Clearly, if the psychiatrist regularly comes to the GP's surgery, this type of consultation is made much easier, but is not essential.

One of the positions that is most jealously guarded by GPs is that of being an independent contractor. It is right and proper for the GP, as the gatekeeper to the portals of specialist care, to be unfettered in choosing treatments and practitioners to whom they wish to make referrals. If the GP feels confident that a few sessions with the community psychiatric nurse is necessary for a selected patient, it is both inefficient and inappropriate for the GP to have to make this referral through the psychiatrist as an intermediary. There is no need for a transfer of medical care and the delay involving a psychiatrist as middleman is unacceptable. Parallels could be drawn with many similar situations in general practice: the ordering of an X-ray, the access to physiotherapy services, and the prescription of a drug which is only available from a hospital pharmacy for individual consultant teams.

The GP is also sometimes concerned about the expansionary nature of some psychiatric services, which appear to want to take over much mental health care in general practice. If this were allowed to happen it could lead to fragmentation of services in primary care (Horder, 1988), developing in time to each medical discipline appropriating part of the service and so denying the GP the position of primary doctor to the patient. The trend towards tight sectorisation of psychiatric services is also viewed with some alarm. If the GP has only one psychiatric team to refer to and, for various reasons, this team is not considered to be appropriate for many of the patients considered for referral, the status of the GP as an independent contractor is lost. He/she has no alternative but to refer to the psychiatric team if further psychiatric care is needed. Although there are exceptions, as for example when a patient happens to come into an unusual category which allows the district services as a whole to become involved (e.g. child psychiatry, forensic psychiatry), the GP's options are too limited.

One of the few recent reforms to the National Health Service to receive almost universal approval is the separation of those wishing to obtain medical service (the purchasers) from those delivering these services (the providers), and this is likely to persist irrespective of the political complexion of succeeding governments. The GP is in the almost ideal position as a purchaser, with direct knowledge of the medical needs of the population and the ability of the services to satisfy them. We cannot give increased powers to GPs and other purchasers and yet continue with restrictions imposed by catchment areas which limit the choice of provider to just two, or in other places to no choice at all.

In any case, GPs as a group are now confident enough to make informed clinical decisions about most of the patients with mental health problems. Many want to develop their services for these patients without the need for secondary care and, if in so doing the psychiatric services have to give up part of their resources, this ought to be accepted. Not only may such expansion of primary care be an advantage for patient care but it will also reduce demands on specialist psychiatric care. There are some who feel that the GP is so much better placed to offer comprehensive care to patients with mental illness than the psychiatrist that almost all the resources currently attached to the community parts of psychiatric services should be redirected to primary care, where it could be used more wisely.

The view from outside the professions

The opinions of psychiatric patients have been traditionally regarded as unimportant in the planning of psychiatric services. Psychiatric patients have always seemed to have a lower status than those with other disorders and we need to be reminded that we have only recently shaken off the notion that mental illness was a synonym for a group of degenerative conditions that placed its sufferers apart from other people in society. There has also been a long-standing paternalistic attitude towards psychiatric patients, often well intentioned but generally assuming that other people know best what is good for them.

   This assumes that all patients both are less able to deal with decisions about their lives and have impaired judgement about the choices open to them. Thus it is therefore necessary for psychiatrists and other professionals to act on patients' behalf and act, in effect, in loco parentis. This of course finds its greatest expression in the operation of the Mental Health Act, under which psychiatrists and social workers can take decisions on behalf of patients and, in particular, can treat them in hospital against their will. Mental health professionals as a consequence were often more feared than respected by patients, and if one or two had the temerity to offer their own opinions they were patted on the head, ever so gently, and asked to go and occupy their little heads with more important things.

   Much has changed in the last few years. It has become recognised that patients with mental health problems have an important part to play in their own treatment. At least they need much more information about their treatments with some attempt at collaboration so that compliance is improved; at best their views about management are obtained before a treatment strategy is developed and the patient is one of the owners of that strategy, not a passive participant. This applies to all psychiatric illness, not just the 'minor' end of the spectrum where patients' complaints are said to be 'reality based', and thereby differentiated from those with more serious (psychotic) illness. The consumer society has been slow to penetrate the field of mental health but is now firmly established.

Now that the patients, and their carers, have a better knowledge of the different approaches available in the treatment of mental illness they are able to come to some conclusions about their preferences. It is all very well psychiatrists saying that the only effective treatment for a major illness such as schizophrenia is antipsychotic drug therapy and that in 'controlled trials' all other approaches are less effective, but psychiatrists do not have to suffer the restlessness of akathisia, the restrictions of Parkinsonian symptoms, and the awful movements of tardive dyskinesia. Similarly, their carers are no longer satisfied with decisions made without their involvement, such as 'community care is best', when that care consists of merely dumping the patient on their next of kin, the local authority or housing agency, and asking them to cope as best they can.

There has been a definite shift in the balance towards consumers of mental health services. Initially their interests were represented mainly through mental health charities, of which MIND is the best-known in the UK. MIND has an excellent record of campaigning for patients' rights, and although appearing at times to have little influence, it has been David toppling the Goliath of the mental health system on many occasions. Its success has led to the growth of other mental health charities with whom carers, often the relatives, of psychiatric patients often play the most prominent role. These include MENCAP, the National Schizophrenia Fellowship, and SANE. In each of these, the views of the patients are being articulated mainly by people who know them extremely well, but these organisations also reflect the opinions of other professionals and voluntary agencies involved with mental health care. The achievements of this lobby have been impressive, perhaps most clearly in the revision of the Mental Health Act in 1983, which gave much greater expression to patients' rights than the previous Act of 1959.

More recently, patients themselves have shown that they have a voice independent of their carers and advocates. This has now become an active issue in the UK largely because of changes that have taken place in Holland over the past ten years. In 1981, the Patients' Advocates Foundation (PVP) was founded in Holland as an independent organisation to help patients in pursuing their complaints, to give advice on their legal rights, and to liaise with mental health services over implementing change on behalf of patients. The success of this enterprise has been reinforced by the establishment of patients' councils within psychiatric hospitals over the past 20 years.

Similar user councils have now been established in many cities in the UK, including London, Nottingham, Sheffield, Leeds and Newcastle. User advocacy is under discussion in most of the health districts in the country (Barker & Peck, 1988) and funding is being made available to extend its development.

Although users as part of their mental illness may hold bizarre opinions, there is a danger that professionals in the mental health services will fail to take their complaints as seriously as if the same views were expressed by a 'normal' person. There is also a fear that many of the organisations for mental health users are determined to overthrow existing mental health structures and replace them with something new and untried. The members of these organisations do not regard themselves as users but as survivors, who view treatment received by mental health professionals as controlling and largely negative in content. If the professionals do not listen to the genuine concerns of their patients they will find themselves facing a movement that is not in the business of compromise.

Many professionals in the mental health services sympathise with these opinions and, by supporting them, make it clear that they contain important ideas. In articulating this support they are attempting to move the balance of psychiatric care from a controlling system that is often acting more on behalf of society than for patients themselves, to a genuine collaborative enterprise. In the words of one of their supporters:

> "what is needed is a philosophy and an approach that is aware of its own values and assumptions, makes them explicit to the client, offers the client a choice as to whether he or she agrees with or wishes to act on those values or assumptions, and makes the necessary support available if the answer is yes." (Johnstone, 1989, p. 289)

The user movement is not just a passing whim but a powerful force that cannot be ignored by anyone in the mental health services.

3 Meeting the need

There are many ways in which the need for increased attention to mental health problems in primary care has been perceived. In this chapter we discuss them again from the three separate standpoints of the psychiatric services, the GP and other primary care services, and the voluntary sector and other professionals. As already noted, there are important differences between their approaches because each focuses on a different part of the population seen in primary care.

The psychiatric view: liaison psychiatry in general practice

Until the late 1950s psychiatric services were almost entirely based on mental hospitals. Contact between primary care and psychiatric services was through the written word for 'cold' referrals such as those to out-patient clinics, and by telephone for emergencies, usually those requiring emergency admission. Face-to-face contact was rare and largely confined to domiciliary visits requested by GPs to consultants for a select group of patients who were difficult to evaluate and for whom the GP was unable to come to a firm conclusion about the best means of treatment. Domiciliary visits were not considered to be part of everyday practice and, as such, they attracted a special fee for the psychiatrist. This somewhat curious anomaly has continued to the present day, even though psychiatric practice has changed considerably in the meantime.

Then psychiatry discovered community care. This was not a sudden revelation experienced by the profession, like Paul on the road to Damascus, but rather the consequence of a gradually increasing awareness that it was pointless trying to practise community psychiatry without bringing the main deliverer of community psychiatry, the GP, into the planning and delivery of psychiatric services. Liaison psychiatry in general practice was therefore born, but as it remained largely hidden from general view, the more prominent and publicised form of liaison, that between psychiatrists and physicians in general hospitals, appropriated the title 'liaison psychiatry' and this description has become attached so firmly it cannot be applied to the general practice variety without causing some confusion.

The nature of the liaison showed tremendous variation that was determined primarily by the orientation and attitudes of the individual psychiatrists. Psychotherapists were particularly impressed by the development of the new discipline of psychotherapy in general practice stimulated by Michael Balint in the 1950s and 1960s (Balint *et al*, 1972). Group sessions between the psychiatrist and interested GPs in which difficult dynamic problems were discussed therefore became one of the key elements of liaison for these individuals (Mitchell, 1983, 1985). However, it quickly became apparent that this type of liaison could involve only a very small proportion of patients needing psychiatric care and other methods were introduced to widen the scope of liaison. The most obvious one was that of seeing patients referred to the psychiatrist in general practice in the form of regular clinics.

This approach, which subsequently became labelled as the 'shifted out-patient clinic' (Williams & Clare, 1981), covered a wide range of patients. It did not include what Williams & Clare termed the 'liaison attachment model', for example where patients are specially chosen to be seen in the GP's surgery because the psychiatrist or the GP thinks that joint discussion about a treatment plan is necessary. More commonly, the psychiatrist literally 'shifted' his/her ordinary out-patient clinic in the psychiatric hospital to premises set aside at the GP's surgery or health centre. The psychiatrist never saw the GP and the advantage of proximity was rarely capitalised upon. However, complete absence of contact was rare and there was usually some face-to-face contact between GPs and psychiatrists during these regular treatment sessions, albeit of short duration, with most contacts lasting less than five minutes (Darling & Tyrer, 1990).

Yet another group of psychiatrists and interested GPs relied on a primarily educational approach. Regular meetings were held, usually in the primary care setting, where psychiatrists discussed psychiatric issues of mutual interest to both professions, sometimes developing around individual cases as well as on more obvious specialist subjects within psychiatry. This type of interchange uses 'liaison psychiatry' in its fullest sense and is more economical of resources than other models (Creed & Marks, 1989).

Encouraging GPs to refer more patients to psychiatrists was considered during the halcyon days of the 1960s, although it was never formally put forward as a viable model of care. This approach, sometimes called the 'replacement model' (Williams & Clare, 1981), was rejected as uneconomic as it would involve the training of a large number of additional psychiatrists.

Thus psychiatrists had a number of approaches to choose from in the 1980s. In practice, as Williams & Clare themselves predicted, only the liaison attachment model, in its many different forms (Creed & Marks, 1989; Tyrer *et al*, 1990a), was viable. This model, in its various forms, is now practised to some extent by between one in three and one in five of all psychiatrists (Strathdee & Williams, 1983; Strathdee, 1987; Pullen & Yellowlees, 1988).

Although much of the attention has been focused on general adult psychiatry in these developments, other disciplines have also been involved to some extent. Psychogeriatrics was one of the first disciplines to realise the importance of not only seeing people in their homes or in primary care but also trying to treat them there (Jolley & Arie, 1978; Pitt, 1980). This approach naturally led to much greater contact with GPs, although this was not usually accompanied by the setting up of separate clinics in old age psychiatry in general practice; a good secretary involved in liaison with the many disciplines is considered of prime importance. The growth of community teams devoted to specialist subjects, such as substance misuse (particularly alcohol), forensic psychiatry, and family therapy, also encourages greater liaison between the psychiatric services and primary care.

These services have grown in a haphazard fashion and there has been no evidence that any of them has been systematically planned. Much has depended on individual personal relationships between psychiatrists and GPs, the geographical advantages in having primary care clinics in areas of lower population and of large area, and professional attitudes about community psychiatry.

Although it is difficult to find any common philosophy behind these developments, at least some of the elements followed from the notion that mental illness could be treated more effectively if it was detected at an early stage. The practice of 'crisis intervention' in psychiatry developed from the pioneering work of Caplan (1964), but in a very different setting from that of general practice in the UK. Caplan, when working in child psychiatry in Israel, realised that the transfer of children to hospital was a far from ideal way of dealing with psychiatric disturbance, and that it was much better both to anticipate the disturbance wherever possible and to treat it at home. It is interesting that this view of child psychiatry has now prevailed to such an extent that very few patients with childhood psychiatric disorders are now admitted to hospital, although the corollary of treating most of them at home has not been followed, since so many present their problems in the GP's surgery (Bailey & Garralda, 1989). Caplan's approach was essentially a preventive one. This included: primary prevention, the ability to increase natural resistance to mental disorder by improving adaptive functions; secondary prevention, the detection of the first signs of mental illness so that early treatment would be implemented; and tertiary prevention, intervention to reduce the handicapping effects of mental disorder or its recurrence.

Although primary prevention remains an elusive goal in psychiatry (Newton, 1988) and there are few who can claim to have demonstrated it, the secondary and tertiary varieties have been practised to varying degrees over the past 30 years. Nevertheless, the benefit in public health terms has been extremely limited (Holland & Fitzsimons, 1990), suggesting either that the research evidence is overstated or that its application to practice has been delayed, prevented, or ignored.

Crisis intervention remains an active principle in community psychiatry and in one part of the country, the London Borough of Barnet, it has been a central component of the psychiatric services for nearly 20 years. The aim of such intervention is to make as many resources available to treat the problem at the time of crisis because at these times people are most receptive to change. If the intervention is appropriate then the pathways to restitution can be developed early and the services withdrawn at an early stage.

Although GPs are not conceived to be an essential element of crisis intervention, they cannot escape being involved in this exercise and often can become key movers. However, even when crisis intervention is not formally practised, the idea of seeing patients early in primary care, before they have had a chance to develop more maladaptive behaviour or other symptoms that make them less receptive to change, is implied in much of the growth of liaison psychiatry in general practice. The intervention takes place at the GP's surgery, and although this may not be as desirable as the patient's home for those who propose crisis intervention, it is nonetheless superior to the psychiatric hospital, where most psychiatric patients feel extremely vulnerable. The primary care setting is usually well known to the patient and is perceived as much less threatening than the psychiatric unit, and this helps assessment of mental health problems.

The notion that intervention at an earlier stage than might otherwise be the case, at a place that is at least neutral in that it is known to both psychiatrist and patient but is the home base of neither, and the opportunity for treatment to be given in such a way that the patient continues to live at home, are all powerful components of both primary care psychiatry and crisis intervention. Unfortunately, the crisis intervention model has not been shown to be the preferred option for psychiatric services as a whole and there are no satisfactory research studies that demonstrate its superiority over alternatives. The same can be said of general practice psychiatry, because evidence such as reduced use of hospital beds (e.g. Tyrer *et al*, 1984) is not necessarily an indication of a superior service. Nonetheless, there is no evidence that shifting more resources into primary care psychiatry results in patients being less well than when seen in the more conventional hospital service (Ferguson *et al*, 1992), and there is a great deal of supporting evidence that it is preferred by patients and GPs to a hospital-orientated model (Tyrer, 1984; Goldberg & Huxley, 1992).

General practice initiatives

Although much of the published research concerned with the expansion of hospital psychiatry into primary care has come from psychiatrists, this should not imply that the GP has not been equally active in developing this service. There have also been some separate initiatives in which psychiatric resources have been brought into primary care by the GP.

One of the most marked has been the referral of patients to community nurses direct from primary care without the intervention of psychiatrists. In such cases the GP has a clear notion of what is needed for the patient and wishes to maintain continued medical responsibility. Most of these patients suffer from one of the neurotic disorders and the type of treatment is usually a psychological one, particularly anxiety management and relaxation training, and behaviour therapy for phobic disorders. The new treatment of cognitive therapy is also assuming increasing importance in this field.

Direct referral of patients from general practice to community psychiatric nurses is becoming increasingly common. In 1985 community psychiatric nurses nationally received 23% of their referrals from GPs, but by 1990 this proportion had increased to 36% (compared with 43% from psychiatrists) (White, 1991, p. 25). If the trend continues, by the year 1995 the GP will be the main referral agency to the community psychiatric nursing services. Indeed this had already happened in 1990 in several regions of the UK (Northern, Trent, South East Thames, Oxford, and South Western Regions).

This approach is preferred by GPs because it is more efficient, as it misses out the unnecessary middleman of the consultant psychiatrist, gives the GP more control of treatment, and continuity of care is maintained. Community psychiatric nurses are also satisfied, because it gives them the opportunity for acting with greater independence in treatment areas for which they have already received special training. Many community psychiatric nurses have completed courses organised through the English Nursing Board which enable them to take on this wider role, and there is a feeling that their psychiatric colleagues are not as aware of these skills as they ought to be. Too many psychiatrists seem to regard such nurses as an army of mobile injection administrators for chronic psychiatric patients, mainly with schizophrenia. The opportunity to deal with a fellow professional, a GP, as an equal, and the gratifying response that many of the patients make to treatment, encourages this type of collaboration.

Psychologists have also been involved frequently in direct referrals from primary care and in many parts of the UK psychologists work more closely with their GP colleagues than with their psychiatric ones. As with the community nurses, psychologists often feel their special skills are not fully appreciated by their psychiatric colleagues, and particularly in the field of neurotic disorders, where cognitive, psychodynamic and behavioural approaches may reap great benefits, the most appropriate referrals appear to be coming from GPs rather from psychiatrists. In some parts of the UK psychologists have set up liaison clinics in primary care in exactly the same way as their fellow psychiatrists have, but referrals are more selective and treatments more often planned in advance.

Although some psychiatrists are concerned about these developments because GPs appear to be diverting mental health professionals from what the psychiatrists consider to be more important work, this type of criticism is hardly fair if it is based only on professional rivalry. We need to direct our services to where they are needed and where they are most effective, and the GP often has a different view of this from that of the psychiatrist. Of course, a service which is set up solely because it is demanded is not necessarily an effective one, and we need much more evidence before we can decide what is the best use of our resources.

Jarman (1992) has shown that when GPs increase their own mental health services (e.g. by direct referrals to community nurses who visit the surgery regularly, attachment of local authority social workers and welfare rights advisers) this is accompanied by a fall in the numbers of referrals to specialist psychiatric services. Psychiatric services could therefore have another reason for encouraging these developments. If more psychiatric care can be given in general practice it will not just be added to the care given in psychiatric settings, it will replace it.

Another advantage of promoting these developments is that those groups who currently make much less use of the psychiatric services than would be expected from their needs, such as ethnic minorities, are probably more likely to come to their GP for their mental health care, although direct evidence of this is not available. The stigma of the psychiatric clinic remains a real one and there is nothing like the same reluctance to attend the GP's surgery.

If GPs are to take a wider role in managing patients with psychiatric illness in primary care they will need to have good means of assessment. It is a sad reflection on the status of conventional psychiatric classification in general practice that simple descriptive terms are used, such as 'frequent attenders', 'chronic psychosis' and 'fat-folder patients' (those whose records sit like cuckoos in practice surgeries, crushing and pushing aside their slim counterparts of patients who rarely seek advice). New ways of making sense of mental illness in primary care are needed urgently by the GP; the move towards greater control of clinical management and specific referrals will stimulate these developments.

The patient's voice

There is a tradition in psychiatry that the patient has no say in treatment. This developed from the early days of the subject in which the only 'treatment' available was incarceration in squalor, punishment with whips and flails, and an unbelievable range of methods of restraint. It is not surprising that the patient was not asked whether these treatments were acceptable, because almost invariably the answer would have been no, and such responses would have been discounted. Even when more humane methods of treatment evolved in the 19th century, there was still a paternalistic attitude towards the patients that left them in no doubt that they were to be treated but not heard.

Although since the birth of psychological treatments there has been increasing emphasis on collaboration as an essential part of good treatment, all too often the old attitudes persist. In particular, with illnesses which belong to the major psychoses, in which patients' judgement and insight is affected in the acute stage, the assumption is that such patients are unable to make a coherent judgement about their treatment at any time in the course of their condition, and it is up to the doctors and other therapists to decide what would be best for the patient irrespective of the person's wishes.

This view is short-sighted and doomed to failure. The only way in which patients could be forced to cooperate with treatment is to lock them up in secure hospitals and impose Draconian curbs on their personal freedom. At the present day this practice is confined only to a small group of extremely dangerous psychiatric patients; most others spend most of the time outside hospital in varying degrees of independence. If the patient has never been persuaded that the treatment plan decided on his/her behalf is an appropriate one, then cooperation ceases. The psychiatrist often has an interpretation about this lack of cooperation, euphemistically called 'poor compliance', and terms like 'psychopathic' and other unpleasant adjectives such as 'impossible', 'incorrigible', 'difficult', and 'irresponsible' are used to catalogue this behaviour. In fact, if most normal people had to undergo the treatments that have been meted out to the psychiatric patient without any agreement they would have abandoned cooperation long ago, and so it is quite wrong to assume that lack of cooperation is due to some inherent fault in the psyche or part of the major psychiatric illness.

Patients who fail to cooperate often drift to the edges of society and receive little or no care. In recent years their cause has been championed by the growth of user groups representing the interests of psychiatric patients in many countries. This 'user movement' has reached its most highly developed form in Holland, where in every part of the country there are patients' councils which elect users of psychiatric services regularly and play a major part in the treatment policies of hospitals. Those who have attended such meetings have often commented about the extra dimension that is added when users are present at meetings normally peopled only by managers and clinicians. The description of the unpleasantness of symptoms – such as the restlessness produced by antipsychotic drugs (akathisia), the feelings after coming round from electroconvulsive therapy (ECT), and the depth of frustration when a point of view never seems to be heard – have an impact on people's thinking and have led to more humane decisions being reached.

This movement has grown in the UK also, and centres at Nottingham, Chesterfield, Newcastle and other towns have grown in the last five years. Psychiatry in primary care is well placed to cooperate with this movement because it does not carry the stigma of psychiatric hospitals, and GPs, in their neutral position, are considered more a friend than a foe by users. There is a potential for genuine collaboration between the user movements and mental health care, but it is in danger of becoming a relationship characterised by conflict rather than by cooperation (Chamberlin, 1988).

Assessment and treatment in primary care

General practitioners have long been aware, because their service is a reactive one, that those who clamour and complain the most tend to get more service than those who are less forceful. Many patients with mental disorders come into the latter category and we need to have appropriate management systems in primary care which ensure that none of these important groups are neglected. We need to have more sensitive detection of these groups and conditions if we are to treat them appropriately. Considerable success has been achieved in recent years in helping GPs to identify depressive disorders in patients, who do not always present their problems as primarily those of mood. This has been done by improving interviewing skills (Goldberg *et al*, 1980) and by highlighting the important questions which must be asked when patients are being assessed in primary care. Without this increased sensitivity much psychiatric disorder remains undetected. For example, in one study in which independent assessment was made of patients presenting with major depressive disorder, half of them were not recognised as depressed by the GP (Freeling *et al*, 1985). The use of screening instruments such as the General Health Questionnaire (GHQ) may also help to expose hidden psychiatric morbidity (not just depression), which can then be followed up by the GP (Johnstone & Goldberg, 1976).

However, despite some success with depression, which is currently being highlighted in a joint campaign between the Royal Colleges of Psychiatrists and General Practitioners, there is still a great deal of uncertainty about the best way of classifying the psychiatric disorders found most frequently in primary care. The psychiatric classifications of the World Health Organization (ICD) and the American Psychiatric Association (DSM) have been created by psychiatrists for psychiatrists, and are not usually applicable to primary care, not least because they do not lend themselves to therapeutic decisions. Attempts to reform these to take into account social functioning and life circumstances have largely been unsuccessful (Jenkins *et al*, 1988). There are arguments in favour of abandoning the approach that attempts to divide up the distress of psychiatric patients by compartmentalising them into different disorders. Some have advocated a holistic approach that diagnoses people rather than medical or psychiatric conditions and takes into account the individual stresses and circumstances that together create unique problems, each of which needs to be examined afresh (Pietroni, 1988).

Research questions

- Are patients with psychiatric disorders in primary care more likely to be diagnosed correctly and to comply with treatment than those with similar disorders in psychiatric practice?
- Is a classification of psychiatric disorders in primary care based on problem orientation more effective than a classification based on separation into defined 'disorders'?
- Which is the most useful classification of psychiatric disorders for GPs?

Whatever strategy is adopted certain groups deserve special attention, and these are worth discussing individually.

Frequent attenders

These people may appear anomalous, as they frequently come to the attention of GPs and they are not 'shrinking violets' when they put forward their problems. Nevertheless, there is a tendency for all practitioners to dismiss such people with unattractive labels such as 'hypochondriac' or 'personality disorders' without adequate prior assessment. It is good practice for frequent attenders to have their status reviewed regularly and to question openly whether the current approach to treating them is correct; the very fact of frequent attendance suggests that it may not be.

Chronic schizophrenia

Patients when they are in the acute stages of schizophrenia attract attention of society by their bizarre behaviour and often wild delusions and hallucinations. In chronic schizophrenia these features are less prominent and apathy, disinterest and withdrawal replace them. Often the original delusions and hallucinations are still present but they are not acted upon and only expressed to those who are willing to listen. These patients are recognised nationally to be at the top of the list for 'priority services', but in practice this usually means that they are not receiving any form of priority at present and are unlikely to do so unless there is a change in the attitudes and approach of the caring professions. This is now being recognised and addressed, not least in work supported by the Mental Health Foundation (Kendrick *et al*, 1991).

The elderly mentally ill

Old age psychiatry has been ahead of general psychiatry in pioneering home-based assessments and treatment of the elderly mentally ill. For this to work well it is necessary to liaise closely with the primary care services, particularly for conditions such as dementia which deteriorate steadily and create a great burden on their carers. The GP is often in the best position to assess when this burden has become intolerable and a change in care is necessary. The frequent coexistence of physical and mental disorders in the elderly also emphasises the need for good liaison.

The elderly often have difficulty in getting to GPs' surgeries and rely heavily on home treatment from members of the primary care team. In a move towards greater efficiency and 'cost-effectiveness' in primary care these needs, which are expensive ones, must not be ignored.

Children

It is only recently that attention has been drawn to the potential of primary care services to attend to the mental health needs of children and adolescents. Approximately one in four children seen by the GP have a psychiatric disorder, usually with somatic manifestations, and children with overt psychiatric disturbance are much more likely to be frequent attenders in general practice than non-disturbed children (Garralda & Bailey, 1986, 1987).

In practice this means that most children with psychiatric disturbance are seen by the GP or another member of the primary care team, notably the health visitor for very young children. However, being seen and being recognised as psychiatrically disturbed are not equivalent, and as so many of these conditions present in the somatic sphere and are relatively mild, it is not surprising that many of them pass undetected.

The important question is not whether primary care psychiatry should be implemented for children, as this is clearly taking place, but how it should be exercised. The GP and other members of the primary care team are clearly best placed to offer care, as most parents with emotionally disturbed children prefer to take them to the GP's surgery than the psychiatric clinic, and this preference is understandably even more pronounced for those who have somatic complaints.

Although information about the effectiveness of treatment for childhood mental health problems in primary care is limited, there is encouraging evidence from pilot studies to suggest that this setting is preferable for treatment and is regarded positively by parents (Garralda, 1992). It is also important to realise that if intervention at this stage is successful it may prevent psychiatric morbidity in later life (Newton, 1988; Rutter, 1989).

Research questions

- What are the best ways of improving the recognition of psychiatric difficulties in children?
- Are there advantages in child psychiatric services being attached to general practice in the way that general psychiatric services have been in recent years?

Substance abuse

The increase in numbers of patients abusing 'hard' drugs (heroin, other opiates, cocaine, etc.), 'soft' drugs (amphetamines, cannabis, benzodiazepine tranquillisers, etc.), and solvents is alarming, and all GPs, even in the more 'respectable' parts of the UK, are liable to come across patients suffering from the psychiatric sequelae of these, in addition to the more acceptable social evil of alcohol. We need much better detection of abuse in primary care in order to prevent inappropriate treatment and unnecessary investigations. Screening methods for detecting drugs need to be available in all primary care facilities. The well described connection between intravenous drug users and the spread of HIV/AIDS emphasises the preventive aspect of identifying these patients early and providing a coordinated system of care. The growth of community drug and alcohol teams liaising with general practice is likely to have an impact here.

The homeless mentally ill

Being homeless is similar to being a stateless refugee. With no address it is difficult to obtain benefits and receive other forms of welfare, including medical care. Many services are now geared to 'catchment areas' where people live and, when bureaucracy takes control in these settings, people who are homeless are inconvenient and it is easier to deny their existence.

This would not matter too much if the homeless were intentionally in this state and needed lesser levels of welfare and care than other groups. In fact, as many studies have shown (Lodge-Patch, 1971; Priest, 1976; Timms & Fry, 1989), the proportion of the homeless who are mentally ill is between 35% and 50%. This population is therefore in much greater need than the equivalent housed population. Primary care needs to open its doors to this needy group and take on their care, even if only temporarily. The same applies to those who are not technically homeless but who have been temporarily placed in bed-and-breakfast hotels and similar (largely unsatisfactory) accommodation. In particular, families with young children are particularly vulnerable in such settings to intolerable stresses created by inadequate living conditions, and mental health care often needs to be delivered to the whole family.

Somatisers

This group, consisting of people who express their emotional difficulties in the form of somatic complaints, is one of the most frequently encountered in primary care (Bridges & Goldberg, 1985) and yet one of the most difficult to manage. Put simply, these people do not want to see any professional concerned with the mental health services because they are convinced that their problems are not psychological but physical. They therefore consider a referral to a mental health professional as misplaced and react accordingly. The GP, as the gatekeeper to all medical services, is an acceptable person to consult but, if he/she fails to identify the patient's symptoms correctly, an unending round of needless investigations and consultations may follow in many general hospital departments before it is realised that there is no serious physical pathology.

We urgently need a strategy for investigating these people in primary care; liaison with psychiatric services needs to be done discreetly (if at all) and almost all care will take place in general practice.

Management of change in general practice

There is much reform going on in primary care at present. In spite of evidence from such projects as the Camberwell Primary Care Project (Morley *et al*, 1991), a large part of this has been generated from government independently from professionals in primary care, and economic performance is one of the driving forces behind them. Every practice needs to have its own business plan and the needs of the mentally ill are sometimes seen to be obstacles to the smooth operation of such plans. In planning services in general practice, auditing their effectiveness and evaluating their outcome, it is important that the mentally ill are not forgotten or made to feel unwanted.

There is much to be said for grasping the opportunity offered by the dramatic developments in information technology and for resource directories to be established of the different agencies available for the care of the mentally ill. By involving these more in primary care, an integrated service can be developed that allows the GP to be part of a coordinated team in which the amount of GP involvement with the patients need not necessarily be great. There also needs to be a re-evaluation of the responsibilities of each member of the primary care team with regard to the care of the mentally ill. Psychiatry has discovered many of the advantages of working in a multidisciplinary team; some GPs have not been so keen to embrace it in their own practices. Yet such working would be necessary to cope with the demands of the mentally ill in primary care; they often need considerable input and this could not always be given by even the most dedicated individual GP.

Good information systems will also help to monitor those who are chronically mentally ill and who are poor attenders in general practice. The GP is in the best position to monitor the progress of such people and to ring the alarm bells when contact is lost. The growth of registers of vulnerable patients could encompass primary care, and it is likely in such a system that the GP would be the key worker for many patients.

Research questions
- Is it economic for general practices to continue providing care for the long-term mentally ill?
- Which aspects of mental health care should be provided by the GP personally and which by other members of the primary care team?
- Does a register of vulnerable psychiatric patients in primary care have benefits in management?

Referral to psychiatric services

There remains a conflict between general practice and psychiatry over the most appropriate form of specialist care for patients referred from general practice. There are two main approaches which are being followed, one which can be termed 'contract care' (to acknowledge the new purchasing power of GPs) and the other, preferred by psychiatrists, which can be described as 'reinforcing primary care psychiatry'.

Contract care

General practitioners are in the process of negotiating contracts for all their patients. Many would like to tighten up the contract arrangements for mental health services, which at present are regarded as a core service for which 'block contracts' are made, with few specific requirements. There is no point in being a purchaser of a service unless your views are heard and can influence the provision of that service.

What GPs would like to have is a set of clear care packages available to them so that they can purchase those that they perceive to be valuable and ignore those that are not. In particular, GPs would like to have their increased skills in recognising and assessing mental illness acknowledged so that their opinions are accepted without further assessment by mental health professionals and their decisions regarded as equally informed.

There are many packages that would be purchased with enthusiasm. These include crisis intervention for difficult problems that present unexpectedly in the course of daily work and which require more man-hours and expertise than are available from the primary care team, sessions of behaviour therapy, cognitive therapy and psychotherapy from psychologists, similar sessional commitment from community psychiatric nurses for counselling and other therapies, such as psychological treatments for substance abuse and tranquilliser withdrawal, as well as more conventional referrals to psychiatric out-patient departments.

Such contracts would have clear conditions. For example, crisis intervention would have to be delivered within a specific time from referral, and it may be necessary to set targets for psychological treatments so that outcome can be measured. The GP would be in an ideal position to assess both the immediate and longer-term outcome of treatment, so that informed decisions can be made about future purchases.

If GPs use contract care, they retain a measure of responsibility for the patient, and this includes medical responsibility when no other doctor is involved in the contract. They will retain a monitoring role and be able to purchase new contracts or cancel old ones on the basis of performance. This, GPs will argue, is the most flexible and appropriate way of providing the specialist care required while still retaining close links with primary care.

Reinforcing primary care psychiatry

Psychiatrists are wedded to catchment areas and see the primary care team as a valuable resource that can help to obviate the need for specialist referral to a different site. They would seek to reinforce the skills of the primary care team in dealing with mental health problems. This usually includes the implicit notion that the psychiatric teams are better able to judge what is needed than the GP. Psychiatric teams therefore wish to employ most of their community care personnel, including community nurses, social workers, occupational therapists and psychologists, and to deploy them where the service judges to be most fitting. To allow GPs access to these valuable resources, particularly when they are not seen in the context of a comprehensive service for an area, will lead to conflict because there is a danger that the GP will be seen as 'stealing' resources from patients who need them more.

Thus, for example, a GP who is keen on devoting more out of his resources to mental health care could purchase a large number of sessions of counselling and other psychological treatments from a health authority and give much extra work to community nurses. If the community nurses are employed on this work at the expense of looking after the more seriously mentally ill, who may not figure very highly on the GP's work load, the long-term mentally ill (as is usually the case) will suffer because their 'purchasing power' appears to be less.

A counter-argument may be equally valid. A general practice that is receiving a poor service from its local psychiatric team and feels that it is not using its resources appropriately should have the opportunity of purchasing these resources directly from the practitioners that it wants. By going through the psychiatrist, the GP loses any control over the personnel involved in the care as well as having no direct influence on the treatment offered. As in any customer–provider relationship, the GP would like to have a much greater say in deciding whether the care that is offered is appropriate, particularly when he/she as the customer has expressed a clear preference for one approach or another.

There is plenty of opportunity for compromise between the two models. At present most of the arrangements in primary care belong to the reinforcement model, but contract care is likely to become the norm in many places if government reforms are encouraged to develop further.

Research questions
- Is the GP or the psychiatric team more successful in taking the main clinical responsibility for the long-term mentally ill?
- Do psychologists and community psychiatric nurses working in an open referral system judge that more appropriate referrals come from the GP or the psychiatrist?
- Is it more effective for resources to be allocated to the large number of patients with neurotic disorder in primary care or to the smaller number of those with psychotic disorders?

Training and education

Whenever different disciplines join forces, people become aware that many skills assumed to be universal are possessed only by one group. Although it is not easy to construct a comprehensive 'shopping list' of skills that need to be available to both primary care and psychiatric teams, and which are currently lacking in one or more, we also need to remind ourselves that the GP is primarily a generalist, not a specialist, and he/she cannot be expected to be an expert in all disciplines. Nevertheless, the following list is a suggested start.

Skills usually present in psychiatric teams but lacking in primary care

Diagnosis of psychiatric disorders (e.g. ICD–10, DSM–III–R)

Detailed knowledge of drugs mainly used for psychoses (e.g. lithium, clozapine, pimozide)

Practice of psychodynamic psychotherapy

Family therapy

Cognitive therapy

The workings of the Mental Health Act

Some conditions which are prominently the province of psychiatric subspecialties, for example autism (child psychiatry), bulimia nervosa (general psychiatry), polydrug use (addiction services), some uncommon causes of mental handicap such as inherited metabolic deficiencies (biochemistry, genetic counselling), psychiatric disorder after brain trauma (neuropsychiatry). These generally involve a few individuals only and many GPs would not have any patients with these problems on their lists.

Skills normally present in primary care but lacking in psychiatry

Joint care of combined medical and psychiatric disorders

Care in the first year of life

Long-term care of chronic non-psychotic disorders

Adjustment disorders (including many with mixed anxiety and depressive disorders)

Somatisation (somatoform) disorders

Use of the doctor–patient relationship.

The differences in skills depend largely on experience. Psychiatry remains largely an empirical discipline and much good practice is founded on experience rather than teaching or training. But this is not an economical way of learning, and if we can share these experiences we can improve our skills. The comprehensive training programme for GPs is one way of doing this, but other ways of improving the knowledge and skills of consultant psychiatrists and principals in general practice are necessary. The Mental Health Foundation has taken this issue as one of its priorities for its primary care and psychiatry initiative; regional workshops, video teaching and university courses are all under consideration.

4 The way ahead

Psychiatry and general practice have become close associates over the past 20 years. From a relationship which was little more than acquaintance they are now almost cohabiting. The next 20 years seem destined to increase this association and extend the links across all parts of the psychiatric and primary care services. There is sometimes a danger in regarding all these developments as so excellent in themselves that they do not require further evaluation. This is particularly so in mental health, where evaluation is more difficult than in many other disciplines.

Although most people concerned with the mental health and primary care services know what constitutes good practice and can easily recognise it when it appears, it is not sufficient to rely on these perceptions as the sole means of monitoring improvement in mental health care. We need to have targets and reliable ways of measuring our success in reaching them. This is formally recognised in the setting of strategies for health in all industrialised countries. In *The Health of the Nation* (Department of Health, 1991*a*) the government sets out a health strategy which is strong and detailed on some disorders and scanty and weak on others. Thus with diabetes it is considered reasonable to agree targets that reduce blindness due to diabetes by at least a third, reduce limb amputations from diabetic gangrene by at least a half, and reduce the number of people entering end-stage diabetic renal failure by at least a third. No such targets are proposed in mental health; the reasons are worth giving in full:

> "Some progress has been made in developing both needs assessment and appropriate outcome measures for mental health. However, there is at present no straightforward and objective way of describing, aggregating or monitoring outcomes of care, nor any agreement on clear and reliable measures which could confidently be used as proxies for outcome measures. The work which has started in this

area needs to be followed up vigorously to ensure that progress is made. However, in the present state of knowledge it is unrealistic to set health outcome targets for these services." (p. 87)

However, since this was published the Department of Health has set new targets for mental health: the reduction in the total mortality due to suicide by 15% and that for the severely mentally ill by a third by the year 2000 (announced in July 1992). In primary care we already know of several changes that could be implemented to prevent the problems of Mr Omega described in Chapter 1. The mental health section of the Department of Health has recently agreed on nine further targets that are both desirable and attainable and are worth discussing in full. The nine targets proposed can roughly be divided into training, prevention, and practice.

Training

(a) Each district should set up an integrated and multiprofessional staff training and development training programme, focusing on the relationship between primary and secondary care.

At the conference in Windsor it was clear that training for mental health work in primary care should be organised jointly by disciplines, and this includes all the professionals involved in both psychiatry and general practice. Unfortunately, the primary and hospital care services are, in management terms, quite separate, and it is difficult to establish training programmes that cross disciplines.

Nonetheless, it should be quite possible to force a way through the territorial barriers that prevent joint-funded initiatives for training from being established, and the way is open for pilot programmes to determine the best form of training and to whom it should be given. If this is to work, we cannot have training needs decided by the relevant disciplines separately. Joint enterprises need joint planning and joint responsibilities.

In hoping for these developments, a problem needs to be recognised in general practice. All general practices are businesses, comprising employers and employed, and this has been emphasised increasingly in recent years, This is likely to impose restraints on multiprofessional staff training in a way that does not apply to hospital staff, who have separate lines of management for each profession. Nevertheless, there are organisations, such as the Centre for the Advancement of Interprofessional Education in Primary Health and Community Care (CAIPE) at the Department of Social Science and Administration at the London School of Economics, which have successfully promoted training within the primary care professions and have shown this problem can be overcome.

(b) There should be an integrated training programme organised jointly by health and social services for primary care teams in both the management of crisis and the use of the Mental Health Act.

This is linked to some extent to the previous item but is doubly important because the sound management of crises demands good coordination and awareness of others' skills. There has already been a wealth of experience accumulated in many parts of the UK through the operation of crisis intervention teams, but little evidence that they are superior to other forms of care, including related approaches involving early intervention. Yet these approaches have the merit of common sense; a large proportion of psychiatric problems present as emergencies and if they are tackled quickly and on the spot it is reasonable to expect that they would be better treated.

Something is wrong here; crisis intervention is perceived by GPs and carers in particular as an important psychiatric service, yet it remains an idiosyncratic minority in most psychiatric services. Is this because it is clinically ineffective compared with other approaches, because it has low cost-effectiveness, or because it encourages other parts of the service to abrogate rapid assessment and treatment, knowing that the crisis service will take over these responsibilities? We do not know, mainly because the subject has been borne forth on a wave of enthusiasm with committed exponents who are much keener on practising their craft than evaluating it.

We also need to be more accurate in defining crisis intervention. Exactly what constitutes a crisis is far from clear. An earthquake is certainly, but most crisis intervention teams deal with microcosmic events in families and small units, and the only common feature is immediate response to the request for help, not the nature of the presenting problem (Punukollu, 1991). Unless we can define the scope of these services there is likely to be confusion in both psychiatric and primary care services, which are unlikely to have identical views on what constitutes a crisis.

The importance of this subject is recognised by the recent appointment of Dr André Tylee (St George's Hospital) at the Royal College of General Practitioners as Senior Mental Education Fellow, funded by the Mental Health Foundation as well as by the Department of Health and the Gatsby Foundation. Unless we have a common language we shall have difficulty in 'teaching the teachers'. The content of training is crucial, and within the next two years the results of this investment and the results of pilot studies should be available to form the substance of a training strategy.

(c) Each general practice should identify one member of the team to take special responsibility or interest in mental health, who would ensure continued training for other team members.

This recommendation has already been adopted in many of the larger group practices in which some specialisation has been in operation for many years. If one member of the practice is particulary interested in mental health matters then it is eminently sensible for this person to take on the educational responsibility for training in all aspects of the subject. This of course needs to be accompanied by similar educational responsibility for other parts of medicine, so that no subject is neglected. For smaller general practices this recommendation is much more difficult to achieve. However, with the growth in numbers of practice nurses and counsellors it is not only appropriate but necessary to expand the multidisciplinary involvement in primary care so that these other disciplines take on responsibilities for training at least as much as GPs. The roles of these new workers need to be evaluated as they will not all develop equal skills, but there are exciting possibilities ahead.

If we do this well there should be a core element of knowledge in each general practice that is largely independent of professional discipline. Medical responsibility will remain with the GP, but the increasing dissemination of skills in psychological treatments makes it likely that counsellors, practice nurses and health visitors will be the chief repositories of these skills in many practices. The GP will continue to have a key role in determining whether patients need further medical intervention and to take decisions about the most appropriate course of action for those who present with complaints that could have primary medical or psychiatric causes (e.g. somatic symptoms).

Multiprofessional practice-based training is supported strongly by the Royal College of General Practitioners, and in many regions it is possible for GPs to obtain postgraduate training allowance credits for carrying out this work. There is no reason why this arrangement should not become universal. A start has been made with a joint project by King's College School of Medicine and Dentistry and the Open University. This aims to improve the skills of workers in primary care and promote distance learning for people in general. The Royal Colleges of General Practitioners and Psychiatrists have also recently agreed a joint statement on the psychiatric content of vocational training for general practice, so collaboration is developing on several fronts.

(d) There should be vocational training and continued education of GPs and other primary care staff about risk factors for depression, suicide, drug abuse and dependence, and relapse in major psychoses.

Risk factors are important but can sometimes be a snare, as many initiatives in medicine to anticipate illness through recognition of risk (a good example is the dietary consumption of cholesterol) have proved useless. Nevertheless, in the mental health services there are clear populations who are at greater risk, and we need to identify them and at least attempt to focus our services on them.

At present most of the services in primary care for patients with mental illness are reactive in nature. Like Alice in *Through the Looking-glass,* we appear to be running as fast as possible to remain in the same place. Patients present with unpleasant symptoms for which they want immediate relief. The GP's reputation depends much more on the ability to relieve these symptoms quickly than on preventing their recurrence by judicious proactive intervention. Although the phrase 'prevention is better than cure' is in danger of becoming diminished in its impact through overuse, it still remains apposite, and if staff in primary care are able to prevent episodes of mental illness recurring they will have made an important clinical advance. The shift towards a more proactive approach requires a change in attitudes and education in mental health; it should start in the undergraduate curriculum and be reinforced regularly.

The GP needs to be backed up by other personnel in this task. Counsellors in general practice are not yet the norm but are increasing in number. There is little doubt that such staff can not only provide a valuable service but also reduce the need for specialist referral (Jarman, 1992). What is now needed is research to establish what separates effective counselling from the disparate range of services currently available so that training can be focused accordingly.

(e) Training opportunities in cognitive and behavioural therapies should be expanded for mental health care staff, GPs, practice nurses, and health visitors.

There is sometimes a belief in primary care that almost all psychological treatments are too time consuming to be carried out in primary care. This was certainly true when psychoanalysis was the only treatment available, but in the last 30 years there have many other therapies introduced that require much shorter treatment. Many aspects of cognitive–behavioural therapy can be used effectively in general practice following a thorough functional analysis of the presenting problem. For example, stress and anxiety management techniques and response prevention in obsessive–compulsive disorders can be given within the confines of general practice consultations because their essential elements take only a few minutes to explain and can be reinforced by written instructions, self-help books, and homework between appointments (Mathews *et al,* 1981). The proper application of computer-led therapy also needs evaluation. The newer treatment of cognitive therapy, in which replacement of negative or dysfunctional thoughts with more positive ones is effective (Teasdale *et al,* 1984), can also be shortened to the extent that it can be carried out in primary care, although its effectiveness compared with other forms of treatment remains untested (Kelly & France, 1987). The role of practice nurses and counsellors may also be important in these therapies; to date, psychologists and psychiatrists have been the prime movers.

There are many advantages in these skills being drawn into primary care. Treatment remains within the general practice, there are no referral delays to specialist services, and there is better continuity of care.

Research questions
- Do general practices that have some specialisation in mental health refer fewer or more patients to the psychiatric services than others?
- Can GPs prevent recurrent depression?
- What are the essential ingredients of good counselling?

Prevention

(f) All patients with severe mental illness should be registered with a GP, receive annual physical health checks, and some health education.

This recommendation reflects the fact that those with mental morbidity also have more physical morbidity than the average person. Although annual health checks are no longer expected for the population as a whole, the greater risk in those with mental health problems accounts for this recommendation. It should be possible to reduce preventable deaths by providing health education, and one attainable target is to provide such health education on smoking to 50% of psychiatric patients, particularly those with chronic psychoses, by 1995, and to 90% by the year 2000 (Thornicroft & Strathdee, 1991).

(g) Each GP's surgery should have a practice case register of patients with severe mental illness. This should link in with a centralised case register which would be available in all districts for people with severe, long-term mental health problems.

Although case registers for psychiatric patients have been in existence for many years (and indeed have been stimulated largely through the initiatives of the Department of Health) they have been used primarily for research purposes rather than clinical practice. In order to be of value in clinical practice, case registers need to be easily accessible and kept up to date, so that when patients present to professional staff who do not already know them the staff can quickly be appraised of developments and make appropriate decisions. Unfortunately there has been concern from organisations acting on behalf of the mentally ill that such registers could be used against rather than for patients' welfare. These concerns, mainly involving confidentiality and the dangers of coercion, need to be addressed but this does not mean that the concept of such case registers is wrong. Everyone, no matter what their status in a health service, is a name or a number on a register somewhere. However, before registers spring up like many-headed hydra in health districts, we need to have data on their value and effectiveness. They can be expensive in terms of time and resources, and are sometimes looked on suspiciously as sources of research information rather than aids to clinical practice. Nevertheless, the general principle of such registers is excellent. The most vulnerable psychiatric patients frequently have contact with many different services consecutively, and if such services are not kept abreast of developments they cannot hope to integrate their care. One of the main advantages of having access to information on a case register is that unnecessary referrals are avoided and fragmentation of care, all too common in some forms of severe psychiatric illness, is prevented.

However, at this stage it is unrealistic to expect most practices to be able to set up such registers, although the value of the exercise in planning services for the mentally ill is well demonstrated (e.g. Jarman, 1992). A more ambitious task is to integrate local registers in general practice with district ones in the psychiatric services; with the growth of computer technology, this is certainly feasible.

Research questions
- Would 'well mind' clinics in primary care reduce the incidence of primary care psychiatric disorder?
- Does the practice case register of patients with severe mental illness reduce the incidence of those dropping out from care?

Practice

(h) All primary care practices should have a written mental health policy for detecting and managing mental illness in the practice, for both the common mental disorders and the care of patients with more severe and chronic mental illness.

There remains great variation in the ability of GPs to detect mental illness, and improved training is only one of the ways of combating this. A clear policy available to all in the primary care team might improve the sensitivity of detection of the important psychiatric disorders.

The challenge here is an enormous one and there are no pioneers at present. However, the introduction of audit to all health care is bound to stimulate the development of practice policies as it has done already for conditions such as diabetes and asthma. Such exercises can be relatively simple. For example, the Defeat Depression Campaign of the Royal Colleges of Psychiatrists and General Practitioners to improve the recognition and treatment of depressive illness could form the substance of a written policy for depression in general practice which could be monitored by recording the incidence of attempted and actual suicides.

(i) All local primary and secondary care teams should develop good practice protocols for the management of common psychiatric disorders.

This extends the previous recommendation to a wider professional group. For example, the policy guidelines for the treatment of depression mentioned above could be extended to include the important issue of when to refer a patient to the psychiatric services. There is now sufficient consensus within the profession for such protocols to be developed. The start made by the Royal Colleges of Psychiatrists and General Practitioners can easily be extended to include similar joint recommendations in schizophrenia, anxiety, eating disorders, dementia, and child psychiatry.

Unfortunately this exercise is handicapped by the confusing nomenclature of psychiatric disorders. We oscillate from describing 'diseases' (e.g. schizophrenia, post-traumatic stress disorder) to describing service groupings (e.g. severe mental illness, long-term mental illness), to giving simple lists of presenting difficulties (advocated in problem-orientated medical records, or POMRs). We have to rationalise the use of these different descriptions before we can agree on policy.

In the longer term, these protocols need to be extended to include social services, psychologists, and even the voluntary mental health sector. The importance of links with the social services was emphasised by Griffiths (1988) in his review of community care:

> "the GP should inform the social services authority of possible community care needs of any patients registered with him who seem to have such needs that are not being met and which appear to be unknown to the social services authority." (p. 15)

For this to work well, good liaison is required; mere transfer of information is not enough. A protocol agreed across the community care services would be invaluable. This will be difficult, because at present the differences in opinion between professions make compromise uneasy, but as training improves and interprofessional boundaries become blurred, successful protocols should be developed which enjoy the support of all.

Research questions
- Does the establishment and promotion of a good practice protocol for the management of depressive disorders reduce the incidence of suicide?
- Is it possible to get agreement between GPs on a common protocol for good practice in mental health?
- Can GPs and psychiatrists agree on a common approach to practice for defined psychiatric disorders?

Involving users

The need to involve users of mental health services was emphasised in Chapter 2. Much of the focus of user involvement has been on psychiatric services in hospitals for the severely mentally ill. Primary care could avoid the mistakes made by psychiatric services, who in general have moved reluctantly and unevenly down the road of patient empowerment, by initiating projects to find the best ways of involving users in the psychiatry of primary care.

This initiative might lead to quite a different structure of cooperation. Primary care psychiatry has several advantages over its specialist equivalent in this respect; it is not generally involved in the deprivation of people's liberties by compulsory admission, it does not have the same stigma as psychiatric hospitals, and it is concerned with all forms of health, not just the vexed one of mental health. Whether a structure is needed for mental health issues alone, or whether it might be better combined with one that deals with all disorders in primary care, remains to be determined. But the subject needs to be addressed; it will not go away and if it is ignored it will force its way on to our agenda before too long.

Targets for special groups in primary care

Child psychiatry

Child psychiatry is predominantly practised as an out-patient service and in many districts there is no specific in-patient provision for children. The child mental health services – psychiatrists, clinical psychologists, social workers and other professionals – are well placed to extend their work but still have far to go in improving its influence on primary care. Much is written about prevention in psychiatry but little is delivered; in the case of child psychiatry, the prospects for successful prevention are much greater.

This needs to start before birth by giving greater attention to the prevention of postnatal depression by identifying high-risk groups, and by early treatment when depression does occur in the puerperium. The early years are extremely important in determining future mental health, and emotional problems cannot be ignored in the hope that they are temporary – 'he's just going through a phase' – because they can inflict lasting damage. There is empirical evidence to show that children presenting at the age of three who remain untreated will continue to present with similar problems at the age of eight (Richman *et al*, 1982). Intervention in the form of a voluntary befriending scheme (Homestart) to disadvantaged families with young children has already produced encouraging results (Eyken, 1982) and both behavioural and psycho-therapeutic intervention in children aged 7–12 years produces better adjustment than a control comparison group, at least in the short term (Kolvin *et al*, 1981).

The high prevalence of somatisation in adult patients might also be reduced by tackling the issue in childhood. Better education of parents is needed so that they understand why the disturbed child presents with physical symptoms even when the cause is primarily emotional. This could not only help the children but also give an insight into their parents' own psychological function in a way that inhibits somatisation.

We have a set of indicators that predict poor functioning in society and greater predisposition to both mental state and personality disorders. Such factors include socioeconomic deprivation, the absence of a parent through separation or death in the first 11 years of life, and lack of parental supervision in the early years, and, most significantly, various forms of child abuse. Although changing these involves political and social change as much as psychiatric intervention, there are still opportunities for the health services to intervene early and provide a preventive role.

The primary care services are excellently placed to recognise these problems and refer at a stage when treatment and intervention are more likely to prevent long-term difficulties. The GP, practice nurse and health visitor have close involvement with children in the few months after birth and, in addition to monitoring the physical health of mother and child, are also well placed to observe and monitor parenting skills and the mental health of the family. In helping to provide a comprehensive preventive service it may well be necessary for the psychiatric, primary care and paediatric services to become a collaborative triumvirate. Already the community paediatric services are well developed in many areas and in some cases are separate from the hospital ones. Collaboration between paediatric and psychiatric services therefore seems to be not only natural but inevitable and with their combined skills, provided that they are linked closely to those of the primary care team, pathology or the factors predisposing to it should be detected early and acted upon, if only by earlier referral to child mental health services.

Targets (for the year 2000)
- At least 20% of child psychiatry practice to involve liaison with community paediatric services and/or primary care.
- All child psychiatric services to devote at least a proportion of their resources to primary prevention.
- The incidence of depressive illness following childbirth to be reduced by 10%.

Substance abuse

The growth of drug misuse continues to be such that it can be rightly described as an epidemic. The number of drug abusers in the UK has risen from around 100 per 1000000 in 1980 to 300 per 1000000 ten years later (Department of Health, 1991*b*) and this does not include those who misuse benzodiazepines or related substances.

Drug misusers are often difficult to engage in regular treatment programmes and frequently attend several facilities simultaneously, mainly in the hope of getting additional supplies of drugs. The GP, and other members of the primary care team, are ideally placed to have a central role in the care of such patients, but in most instances this would be difficult to carry out in primary care alone. It is common in most health districts to have specialist facilities for drug abusers, including a consultant psychiatrist with a special interest in the subject and a community drug team. With drug misusers in primary care it is now recommended that "the model of choice for clinical management is shared care with a specialist" (Department of Health) and in this shared care it is essential to establish which doctor is responsible for drug prescribing. For those patients whose primary contact is with the drug dependency services, it is important for the GP to be kept in touch with progress, even if there is no current contact between the primary care team and the patient.

Targets (for the year 2000)
- All districts to have a community drug team linked to a drug dependency service that offers liaison in primary care.
- Fifty per cent of drug misusers to have their clinical management shared between primary care and specialist drug dependence units.

Alcohol

Although alcohol is just as much a substance of misuse as all others it deserves a separate section. This is partly because of the size of the problem (alcohol-related illness is ten times as common as that related to other substance misuse) and also because alcohol is freely and legally available (as are most socially acceptable dangerous drugs, including tobacco). Tackling the problem of alcohol abuse and its precursors, hazardous and harmful drinking, involves much more than the health services, but nonetheless primary care has an important role in both prevention and management. In particular the GP needs to be able to detect the warning signs of alcohol abuse and dependence at an early stage. This not only prevents future suffering but the problem is tackled when there is likely to be a better chance of successful abstinence. One initiative in Scotland (the DRAMS scheme) helps the GP to identify harmful drinking in surgery attenders and effect reduction in consumption. For those with more established addiction to alcohol the road to abstinence is a long and tortuous one, and the GP must be available for support and succour along the route, as well as the specialised services. The growth of community alcohol teams in many areas, who liaise regularly with GPs and other primary care services, is an invaluable aid to management and, as these develop, the skills and ability of primary care teams to take on the care of large numbers of alcohol-dependent patients will be increased.

Targets (for the year 2000)
- For community alcohol teams to be operating effectively in all health districts.
- At least 50% of all alcohol-related disease to have been detected or suspected by the GP before confirmatory diagnosis.

Old age psychiatry

The mean age of every population in Western countries is increasing. In the UK alone the number of people aged 85 and over will have risen by nearly a third, from 865000 in 1991 to 1146000 by the year 2001. As there is a direct correlation between the numbers of sufferers from conditions such as Alzheimer's disease and the numbers of elderly people, the importance of old age psychiatry is bound to increase. This will have an impact on carers also. Data from the General Household Survey in 1988 (Office of Population Censuses and Surveys, 1988) show that approximately one in ten households has a carer looking after a dependant aged 75 or over, and this proportion is likely to increase.

As the incidence of general medical disorders also increases with advancing age, and as the policy of keeping elderly patients for as long as possible in their own familiar settings is helped by improvements in home care, the need for good collaboration between GPs and psychiatrists will become even greater. The GP is increasingly likely to be the first to detect and manage major mental illness in the elderly and to be the key worker in follow-up.

Targets (for the year 2000)
- To identify by screening of at least 90% of all dementias in primary care.
- To draw up a plan for the assessment, management and review of all patients found to have a dementing illness by screening at the age of 75, this plan necessarily integrating psychiatric and primary care components.

Chronic psychoses

This large group, comprising mainly patients with schizophrenia and manic–depressive psychosis (mainly the former), continues to remind professionals in primary and psychiatric care that our community care falls sadly short of an acceptable service. The challenge is an enormous one, for these patients have seldom in the history of psychiatry been well served by their professional carers. They have been exploited, abused or subjected to intolerable restraint in institutional settings, or ignored and neglected in squalor in the community. Such generalisations are always dangerous as all professionals will know of exceptions in which there is a good standard of care and satisfactory quality of life (often provided entirely from the primary care services) and this may sometimes extend to whole services (Johnstone, 1991). However, in the main the neglected or inappropriately placed patients outnumber the ones who are served well, and this remains nothing short of a scandal in an affluent and civilised society.

The challenge here is enormous. Care in hospital is neither clinically appropriate, as these people do not need long-term skilled nursing care, nor personally desirable, as given the choice most of them much prefer being in the community and regard return to hospital as the least desired option (Johnstone, 1991). If community accommodation, either sheltered or independent, and treatment are to succeed, primary care must play a major part. In their survey of GPs, Kendrick *et al* (1991) found that 90% felt that shared care between GP and psychiatric services was desirable for this chronic population, but the best way of delivering and coordinating this remains debatable. In the last resort, however, it appears to be the only realistic option.

In the same survey 83.5% thought that the community psychiatric nurse was the most appropriate key worker for this population, but this may merely follow from the fact that the community psychiatric nurse is the best known of the psychiatric disciplines in primary care. If this suggestion was followed through there would be important changes in the deployment and responsibilities of community nurses. At present they are being asked to take on too many responsibilities and there is a danger that patients with major psychiatric disorders, particularly schizophrenia, will suffer unless they are given priority (Tyrer *et al*, 1990*b*).

It was noted in Chapter 3 that now more than a third of all referrals to community psychiatric nurses are from GPs. The same survey (White, 1991, p. 29) also provided statistics that suggest that patients with chronic mental illness are being bypassed again. Significantly fewer patients with chronic mental illness and schizophrenia were referred to community nurses from GPs than psychiatrists. As there is no evidence that any other professional group is selectively increasing its proportion of referrals with schizophrenia, the increasing march of community nursing towards general practice seems likely to lead to the neglect of these patients.

Targets (for the year 2000)
- To reduce the number of in-patients with psychosis who have been in hospital for over six months and for over one year by 40% (Thornicroft & Strathdee, 1991).
- Ninety per cent of former patients with psychosis to be in contact with services and on a local case register (this ensures that patients are not lost to follow-up as so frequently is the case at present).

Priorities in development

With so many targets to aim for there is a danger that we could fail to see the important bull's-eyes through the forest of arrows! We therefore need to remind ourselves what lies behind these targets and what are their common goals. Despite the definite advances made in mental health assessment and treatment over the past century we are still no nearer to the goal of improving the mental health of the population as a whole. It is possible there have been improvements and we are merely handicapped by our failure to use adequate measures of outcome, as suggested in *The Health of the Nation* (Department of Health, 1991*a*). However, such statistics we do have are not encouraging: suicide rates are rising, not falling, and the prevalence of psychiatric disorder in the community (Table 1, p. 10) is remaining constant.

Although we now place much less reliance on psychiatric institutions in the care of the mentally ill, the reduction in bed occupancy and greater community care has not been accompanied by reduced suicide rates (they are slowly increasing) or reduced readmission rates for chronic or recurring disorders such as the major psychoses. We have also failed to prevent mental illness by earlier intervention.

Why? There are probably many answers, but an important one is that we have concentrated for far too long on the tiny minority of psychiatric patients who come into hospital, hoping, without any real evidence, that if we get this population treated successfully the benefits will slowly percolate to all layers of the services involved with the mentally ill. Now that we are clear that mental illness is, by and large, seen, recognised, treated and followed up in primary care, we have no excuse to neglect this setting. If we can have a small effect on the mental health of the 230 patients per 1000 population presenting each year to primary care, it will have a much greater effect than the continued assault on the 5.7 psychiatric in-patients per 1000.

There is a question all mental health professionals need to ask themselves when seeing and managing a patient: "Is this the best place for me both to assess and to treat this person?" This involves compromise; often assessment requires a quiet clinical setting where there is no disturbance, whereas treatment is often best in the place where there is least disruption to normal life. For patients who are dangerous to others the needs of society also have to be weighed against the benefits to the individual. Nevertheless, in most cases it is easy to detect the places that tend to handicap positive intervention: the busy casualty department for those patients who can find no avenue of help elsewhere, the prison hospital ward for someone who is suicidally depressed, or the acute psychiatric ward for the fearful people who are afraid of going mad.

The pace of developments in medical practice has become ever faster in recent years and we are sometimes lulled into the notion that we merely need to wait for advances to come along and then to implement them accordingly. This idea conveniently overlooks that the application of advance is often much more difficult than its discovery. In mental health the crying need at present is to apply what we already know rather than to know more what to apply. Even if we make no advances of any sort in our treatment of mental illness in the next ten years we have the opportunity to transform prospects for mental health by deploying our resources both when and where they are needed, by ensuring that our therapists possess the necessary skills, that patients are willing participants in our therapies, and that monitoring and required maintenance therapy continue in collaboration for as long as the disorder dictates. These are not trivial aims or unattainable goals; they are within our reach if we can get primary care and psychiatry working in unison.

References

BAILEY, D. & GARRALDA, M.E. (1989) Referrals to child psychiatry. *Journal of Child Psychology and Psychiatry*, **30**, 449–458.

BALINT, M., ORNSTEIN, P.H. & BALINT, E. (1972) *Focal Psychotherapy*. London: Tavistock.

BARKER, I. & PECK, E. (1988) *Power in Strange Places: User Empowerment in the Mental Health Services*. London: Good Practices in Mental Health.

BRIDGES, K. & GOLDBERG, D. (1985) Somatic presentation of DSM–III psychiatric disorders in primary care. *Journal of Psychosomatic Research*, **29**, 563–569.

CAPLAN, G. (1964) *Principles of Preventative Psychiatry*. New York: Basic Books.

CHAMBERLIN, J. (1988) The case for separatism: ex-patient organising in the United States. In *Power in Strange Places: User Empowerment in Mental Health Services* (eds I. Barker & E. Peck), pp. 24–26. London: Good Practices in Mental Health.

CLARE, A.W. & LADER, M. (eds) (1981) *Psychiatry and General Practice*. London: Academic Press.

CREED, F. & MARKS, B. (1989) Liaison psychiatry in general practice: a comparison of a liaison attachment scheme and the shifted out-patient model. *Journal of the Royal College of General Practitioners*, **39**, 514–517.

CROFT-JEFFREYS, C. & WILKINSON, G. (1989) Estimated costs of neurotic disorder in UK general practice 1985. *Psychological Medicine*, **19**, 549–558.

DARLING, C. & TYRER, P. (1990) Brief encounters in general practice: an audit of liaison in general practice psychiatric clinics. *Psychiatric Bulletin*, **14**, 592–594.

DEPARTMENT OF HEALTH (1991*a*) *The Health of the Nation*. London: HMSO.

—— (1991*b*) *Drug Misuse and Dependence: Guidelines on Clinical Management*. London: HMSO.

EYKEN, W., VAN DER (1982) *Homestart: A Four Year Evaluation*. Leicester: Homestart Consultancy.

FAHY, T. J. (1974) Pathways of specialist referral of depressed patients from general practice. *British Journal of Psychiatry*, **124**, 231–239.

FERGUSON, B., COOPER, S., BROTHWELL, J., *et al* (1992) The clinical evaluation of a new community psychiatric service based on general practice psychiatric clinics. *British Journal of Psychiatry*, **160**, 493–497.

FREELING, P., RAO, B. M., PAYKEL, E. S., *et al* (1985) Unrecognized depression in general practice. *British Medical Journal*, **290**, 1880–1883.

GARRALDA, M.E. (1992) Primary care psychiatry. In *Child and Adolescent Psychiatry* (3rd edn) (eds M. Rutter, L. Hersov & E. Taylor). Oxford: Blackwell.

—— & BAILEY, D. (1986) Children with psychiatric disorders in primary care. *Journal of Child Psychology and Psychiatry*, **27**, 611–624.

—— & —— (1987) Psychosomatic aspects of children's consultation in primary care. *European Archives of Psychiatry and Neurological Sciences*, **236**, 319–322.

GATER, R. & GOLDBERG, D. (1991) Pathways to psychiatric care in South Manchester. *British Journal of Psychiatry*, **159**, 90–96.

——, DE ALMEIDA E SOUSA, R., CARAVEO, J., *et al* (1991) The pathways to psychiatric care: a cross-cultural study. *Psychological Medicine*, **21**, 761–774.

GOLDBERG, D. & HUXLEY, P. (1980) *Mental Illness in the Community: The Pathway to Psychiatric Care*. London: Tavistock.

——, STEELE, J. J. & SMITH, C. (1980) Teaching psychiatric interviewing skills to family doctors. *Acta Psychiatrica Scandinavica*, **62**, 41–47.

—— & —— (1992) *Common Mental Disorders: A Biosocial Model*. London:Tavistock/Routledge.

GRIFFITHS, R. (1988) *Community Care: Agenda for Action*. London: HMSO.

HOLLAND, W. & FITZSIMONS, B. (1990) Public health concerns: how can social psychiatry help? In *The Public Health Impact of Mental Disorder* (eds D. Goldberg & D. Tantam), pp. 14–19. Toronto: Hogrefe and Huber.

HORDER, J. (1988) Working with general practitioners. *British Journal of Psychiatry*, **153**, 513–520.

JARMAN, B. (1992) Psychiatric illness and services in a UK health centre. In *Primary Health Care and Psychiatric Epidemiology* (eds B. Cooper & R. Eastwood), pp. 99–108. London: Tavistock/Routledge.

JENKINS, R., SMEETON, N. & SHEPHERD, M. (1988) Classification of mental disorder in primary care. *Psychological Medicine* (monograph suppl. 12).

JOLLEY, D. J. & ARIE, T. (1978) Organization of psychogeriatric services. *British Journal of Psychiatry*, **132**, 1–11

JOHNSTONE, A. & GOLDBERG, D. (1976) Psychiatric screening in general practice. *Lancet, i*, 605–608.

JOHNSTONE, E. C. (1991) Disabilities and circumstances of schizophrenic patients – a follow-up study. *British Journal of Psychiatry*, **159** (suppl. 13).

JOHNSTONE, L. (1989) *Users and Abusers of Psychiatry: A Critical Look at Traditional Psychiatric Practice*. London: Routledge.

KELLY, D. & FRANCE, R. (eds) (1987) *A Practical Handbook for the Treatment of Depression. Are Antidepressants Enough?* Carnforth & Park Ridge: Parthenon.

KENDRICK, T., SIBBALD, B., BURNS, T., *et al* (1991) Role of general practitioners in care of long-term mentally ill patients. *British Medical Journal*, **302**, 508–510.

KOLVIN, I., GARSIDE, R. F., NICOL, A. S. R., *et al* (1981) *Help Starts Here*. London: Tavistock.

LODGE-PATCH, I. C. (1971) Homeless men in London: 1 Demographic findings in a lodging house sample. *British Journal of Psychiatry*, **118**, 313–317.

MATHEWS, A. M., GELDER, M. G. & JOHNSTON, D. W. (1981) *Agoraphobia: Nature and Treatment*. Oxford: Oxford University Press.

MENTAL HEALTH FOUNDATION (1990) *Mental Illness: The Fundamental Facts*. London: MHF.

MITCHELL, A. R. K. (1983) Liaison psychiatry in general practice. *British Journal of Hospital Medicine*, **30**, 100–106.

—— (1985) Psychiatrists in primary health care settings. *British Journal of Psychiatry*, **147**, 371–379.

MORLEY, V., EVANS, T. & HIGGS, R. (1991) *A Case Study in Developing Primary Care: The Camberwell Report*. London: King's Fund.

NEWTON, J. (1988) *Preventing Mental Illness*. London: Routledge and Kegan Paul.

OFFICE OF POPULATION CENSUSES AND SURVEYS (1988) *General Household Survey 1988*. London: HMSO.

ORMEL, J. & GIEL, R. (1990) Medical effects of non-recognition of affective disorders in primary care. In *Psychological Disorders in General Medical Settings* (eds N. Sartorius, D. Goldberg, G. de Girolamo, *et al*). Bern: Huber-Hogrefe.

PIETRONI, P. (1988) Alternative medicine. *Journal of the Royal Society of Arts*, **136**, 791–798.

PITT, B. (1980) Management problems in psychogeriatrics. *British Journal of Hospital Medicine*, **24**, 39–46.

PRIEST, R. G. (1976) The homeless person and the psychiatric services: an Edinburgh survey. *British Journal of Psychiatry*, **128**, 128–136.

PULLEN, I. & YELLOWLEES, A. (1988) Scottish psychiatrists in primary care settings: a silent majority. *British Journal of Psychiatry*, **153**, 663–666.

PUNUKOLLU, N. R. (ed.) (1991) *Recent Advances in Crisis Intervention.* Huddersfield: Institute of Crisis Intervention and Community Psychiatry.

RICHMAN, N., STEVENSON, J. & GRAHAM, P. J. (1982) *Pre-school to School – A Behavioural Study.* London: Academic Press.

RUTTER, M. (1989) Pathways from childhood to adult life. *Journal of Child Psychology and Psychiatry*, **30**, 23–51.

SHEPHERD, M., FISHER, N., KESSEL, N., *et al* (1959) Psychiatric morbidity in an urban practice. *Proceedings of the Royal Society of Medicine*, **52**, 269-274.

——, COOPER, B., BROWN, A. C., *et al* (1966) *Psychiatric Illness in General Practice.* London: Tavistock.

——, WILKINSON, G. & WILLIAMS, P. (1986) *Mental Illness in Primary Care.* London: Tavistock.

STRATHDEE, G. (1987) Primary care–psychiatry interaction: a hospital perspective. *General Hospital Psychiatry*, **9**, 69–77.

—— & WILLIAMS, P. (1983). A survey of psychiatrists in primary care: the silent growth of a new service. *Journal of the Royal College of General Practitioners* **34**, 615–618.

TEASDALE, J. D., FENNELL, M. J. V., HIBBERT, G. A., *et al* (1984) Cognitive therapy for major depressive disorder in primary care. *British Journal of Psychiatry*, **144**, 400–406.

TIMMS, P. W. & FRY, A. H. (1989) Homelessness and mental illness. *Health Trends*, **21**, 70–71.

THORNICROFT, G. & STRATHDEE, G. (1991) The health of the nation: mental health. *British Medical Journal*, **303**, 410–412.

TYRER, P. (1984) Psychiatric clinics in general practice – an extension of community care. *British Journal of Psychiatry*, **145**, 9–14.

—— (1986) What is the role of the psychiatrist in primary care? *Journal of the Royal College of General Practitioners*, **36**, 373–375.

——, SEIVEWRIGHT, N. & WOLLERTON, S. (1984) General practice psychiatric clinics – impact on psychiatric services. *British Journal of Psychiatry*, **145**, 15–19.

——, FERGUSON, B. & WADSWORTH, J. (1990*a*) Liaison psychiatry in general practice: the comprehensive collaborative model. *Acta Psychiatrica Scandinavica*, **81**, 359–363.

——, HAWKSWORTH, J., HOBBS, R., *et al* (1990*b*) The place of the community psychiatric nurse in a comprehensive mental health service. *British Journal of Hospital Medicine*, **43**, 439–442.

WHITE, E. (1991) *The 3rd Quinquennial National Community Psychiatric Nursing Survey.* Manchester: Department of Nursing, University of Manchester.

WILLIAMS, P. & CLARE, A. (1981) Changing patterns of psychiatric care. *British Medical Journal*, **282**, 375–377.

—— & BALESTRIERI, M. (1989) Psychiatric clinics in general practice: do they reduce admissions? *British Journal of Psychiatry*, **154**, 67–71.

WM3OTYR